The Effective Management of Colorectal Cancer

Edited by

David Cunningham MD FRCP
Consultant Medical Oncologist and Head of the GI & Lymphoma Units
The Royal Marsden Hospital, London and Surrey, UK

Daniel Haller MD
Professor of Medicine, University of Pennsylvania Cancer Center
Philadelphia (PA), United States of America

Andrew Miles MSc MPhil PhD
Professor of Public Health Policy and Health Services Research &
UK Key Advances Series Organiser, University of East London, UK

UeL University Centre for
Public Health Policy &
Health Services Research

The Association
of
Cancer Physicians

The Royal College
of
Radiologists

AESCULAPIUS MEDICAL PRESS
LONDON SAN FRANCISCO SYDNEY

Published by

Aesculapius Medical Press (London, San Francisco, Sydney)
Centre for Public Health Policy and Faculty of Science and Health
University of East London
33 Shore Road
London E9 7TA

British Library Cataloguing in Publication Data

A catalogue record for this book is available from the British Library

ISBN 1 903044 07 3

While the advice and information in this book are believed to be true and accurate at the
time of going to press, neither the authors nor the publishers nor the sponsoring institutions
can accept any legal responsibility or liability for any errors or omissions that may be made.
In particular (but without limiting the generality of the preceding disclaimer) every effort has
been made to check drug usages; however, it is possible that errors have been missed.
Furthermore, dosage schedules are constantly being revised and new side-effects recognised.
For these reasons, the reader is strongly urged to consult the drug companies' printed
instructions before administering any of the drugs recommended in this book.

Further copies of this volume are available from:

Claudio Melchiorri
Research Dissemination Fellow
Centre for Public Health Policy and Faculty of Science and Health
University of East London
33 Shore Road
London E9 7TA

Fax: 020 8533 3878

Typeset, printed and bound in Britain
Peter Powell Origination & Print Limited

Contents

Contributors

René Adam MD PhD, Professor of Surgery, Centre Hépato-Biliaire, Hôpital Paul Brousse, Villejuif, France

Fareeda Ahmed MRCP, Department of Oncology, Grampian University Hospitals and University of Aberdeen, Foresterhill, Aberdeen, Scotland

Arie Ariche MD, Centre Hépato-Biliaire, Hôpital Paul Brousse, Villejuif, France

Eli Avisar MD, Centre Hépato-Biliaire, Hôpital Paul Brousse, Villejuif, France

Daniel Azoulay MD PhD, Centre Hépato-Biliaire, Hôpital Paul Brousse, Villejuif, France

Henri Bismuth MD FACS, Professor of Surgery, Centre Hépato-Biliaire, Hôpital Paul Brousse, Villejuif, France

Donald Bissett MD FRCP FRCR, Department of Oncology, Grampian University Hospitals and University of Aberdeen, Foresterhill, Aberdeen, Scotland

Gina Brown MRCP FRCR, Department of Radiology, University Hospital of Wales, Heath Park, Cardiff

Jim Cassidy MD FRCP, Department of Oncology, Grampian University Hospitals and University of Aberdeen, Foresterhill, Aberdeen, Scotland

Denis Castaing MD, Professor of Surgery, Centre Hépato-Biliaire, Hôpital Paul Brousse, Villejuif, France

Alison R Gillams, University College Hospital, London

Daniel Haller MD, Professor of Medicine, University of Pennsylvania Cancer Centre, Philadelphia (PA), USA

Mark Hill MD MRCP, Consultant Medical Oncologist, Gastrointestinal Unit, Department of Medicine, Royal Marsden NHS Trust, Sutton, Surrey

Roger James MRCP FRCR, Director, Cancer Services for Kent, MidKent Healthcare Trust

Sylvie Giachetti MD, Centre de Chronothérapie, Service de Cancérologie, Hôpital Paul Brousse, Villejuif, France

John B Karani FRCR, Consultant Radiologist, Department of Radiology, King's College Hospital, London

Francis Kunstlinger MD, Centre Hépato-Biliaire, Hôpital Paul Brousse, Villejuif, France

William R Lees, Professor of Medical Imaging, University College Hospital, London

Francis Levi MD PhD, Centre de Chronothérapie, Service de Cancérologie, Hôpital Paul Brousse, Villejuif, France

James S McCourtney MD FRCS, Consultant Colorectal Surgeon, Royal Alexandra Hospital, Paisley, Scotland

Howard McLeod PharmD, Department of Oncology, Grampian University Hospitals and University of Aberdeen, Foresterhill, Aberdeen, Scotland

Michele M Marshall MRCP FRCR, Specialist Registrar in Diagnostic Radiology, Department of Radiology, King's College Hospital, London

John MA Northover MS FRCS, Consultant Surgeon, ICRF Colorectal Cancer Unit, St Mark's Hospital, Harrrow, Middlesex

Andreas Polychronis MRCP, Registrar in Medical Oncology, Guy's Hospital, London

David Sebag-Montefiore MBBS FRCP FRCR, Consultant Clinical Oncologist, Yorkshire Centre for Clinical Oncology, Cookridge Hospital, Leeds

Matthew T Seymour MA MD MRCP, Senior Lecturer in Medical Oncology, Cookridge Hospital, Leeds

Kate Sumpter MD MRCP, Gastrointestinal Unit, Department of Medicine, Royal Marsden NHS Trust, Sutton, Surrey

Clare A Topham FRCR, Consultant Clinical Oncologist, St Luke's Cancer Centre, The Royal Surrey County Hospital, Guildford, Surrey

Preface

The paradigms for treatment for colorectal cancer have changed in a major way during the past decade. Colorectal cancer was once considered a surgical disease, whereas now, best clinical practice encompasses the disciplines of clinical genetics, medical oncology, radiotherapy, and, to a lesser extent, molecular biology. The changing shape of treatment is illustrated by the now established role of adjuvant systemic chemotherapy following surgical resections of colorectal cancer, the evolution of combination chemotherapy in the management of metastatic disease and the recognition that patients with metastatic disease may derive longterm benefit from metastasectomy. The role of radiotherapy in rectal cancer has become more clearly defined, although, with more accurate staging methodology, it is hoped that the use of radiation therapy in both the pre- and post-operative setting may be more selective in the future than currently. Surgery remains of key importance in the disease and refinements of techniques such as total mesorectal excision can also improve outcomes in the disease.

In the current age, where doctors and health professionals are increasingly overwhelmed by clinical information, we have aimed to provide a fully current, fully referenced text which is as succinct as possible, but as comprehensive as necessary. Consultants in surgical, medical and clinical oncology and their trainees will find it of particular use as part of their continuing professional development and specialist training, and we advance it explicitly as an excellent tool for these purposes. We anticipate, however, that the book will prove of not inconsiderable use to clinical nurse specialists and oncology pharmacists as a reference text and to commissioners of health services as the basis for discussion and negotiation of health contracts with their practising colleagues.

In conclusion, we thank Sanofi-Synthelabo for the grant of educational sponsorship which helped organise a national symposium held with the Royal College of Radiologists and the Association of Cancer Physicians at the Royal College of Physicians of London, at which synopses of the constituent chapters of this book were presented.

David Cunningham MD FRCP
Daniel Haller MD
Andrew Miles MSc MPhil PhD

PART 1

Evidence and Opinion in Adjuvant Chemotherapy

Adjuvant therapy in colorectal cancer: what constitutes 'best clinical practice'?

Andreas Polychronis and Daniel Haller

Introduction

Colorectal cancer is a leading cause of death in the Western world and is responsible for some 400,000 deaths per year (Pisani *et al.* 1993). Most patients, at presentation, have apparently localised disease. However, the remaining 30 per cent have advanced disease, the majority of whom have distant metastases. Three-quarters of colorectal cancers involve the colon, while the remaining quarter is confined to the rectum, located below the peritoneal reflection. Survival depends on the pathologic staging of the disease, ranging from 90 per cent five-year survival for stage I to less than 5 per cent for stage IV (Fielding 1995). Although a small number of patients with recurrent disease may be cured by salvage resection of their metastases, the majority of colorectal cancer patients with metastatic colon cancer will succumb to their disease. The goal therefore is to identify and remove surgically curable tumours. On the basis of recurrence after potentially curative surgery, and the likely presence of micrometastases, many patients will require some adjuvant treatment programme.

The aim of adjuvant treatment is to target occult viable tumour cells and eradicate them before they become established and refractory to treatment. Important considerations are the risk:benefit ratio of such treatment and achieving a balance between maximum chance of cure or prolonged survival and tolerance of side effects.

In discussing adjuvant therapy one must differentiate between colon and rectal cancers. Rectal tumours in the retroperitoneal location may be more difficult to excise with wide margins and are typically associated with a higher incidence of local relapse than similarly staged colon primary tumors. Adjuvant therapies in stage II and III rectal patients must therefore include approaches, such as more radical resection and radiation, to reduce the risk of recurrence and to improve overall survival.

Adjuvant therapy in colorectal cancer

The initially controversial era of the use of adjuvant chemotherapy in colorectal cancer started over two decades ago, when Li & Ross (1976) suggested an improvement in five-year disease-free survival with single agent 5-fluorouracil (5-FU), post-operatively, in patients with stage II and III colon cancer. The study was criticised for its design (retrospective, non-controlled trial of 89 patients), which failed to take into account differences in patient groups and surgical techniques. The need for prospective, randomised controlled trials (RCTs) emerged.

The first large prospective RCT that demonstrated survival benefit from adjuvant chemotherapy was published in 1988 with the report of the National Surgical Adjuvant Breast and Bowel Project (NSABP) protocol C-01 (Wolmark *et al.* 1988). This compared a post-operative combination of 5-FU, semustine and vincristine to surgery alone, and demonstrated a modest improvement in overall survival of borderline statistical significance. However, several further trials of fluorouracil plus semustine failed to demonstrate a benefit when compared with surgery alone in stage II and III colon cancer, including those conducted by the Southwest Oncology Group and the Italian Colon Cancer Program of the National Research Council (Panettiere *et al.* 1988; Merangolo *et al.* 1989).

A meta-analysis of 17 RCTs of adjuvant chemotherapy in colorectal cancer was performed by Buyse *et al.* in 1989. This showed no statistically significant survival benefit. However, when the analysis was limited to 12 studies using 5-FU-based regimens, a small benefit was suggested (mortality hazard ratio of 0.83 in favour of therapy; 95 per cent confidence intervals, 0.70–0.98). This inconsistency was thought to be due to the heterogeneity of the studies, some with sub-optimal 5-FU administration schedules with varying doses and duration of treatment. When the analysis was further limited to seven studies in which 5-FU was administered for at least one year, a statistically significant benefit to chemotherapy was observed. However, the clinical relevance and statistical superiority of a specific regimen had not been identified.

Following the initial uncertainty as to the effectiveness of standard bolus fluorouracil treatment, other avenues of adjuvant treatment were explored. One of the most controversial interventions included levamisole, an antihelminthic agent. Although its mechanism of action in malignancies is uncertain, it has been thought to function as an immunomodulator, acting synergistically with the antitumour effects of 5-FU, possibly through selective stabilisation of mRNA (AbdAlla *et al.* 1995). In 1978, the North Central Cancer Treatment Group/Mayo Clinic (NCCTG) initiated a randomised trial comparing post-operative levamisole or an empiric combination of fluorouracil and levamisole to surgery alone in stages II and III colon cancer. After a median follow-up of nearly eight years, there were improvements in recurrence-free survival for both treatment arms, which were borderline ($P=0.05$) for levamisole alone but statistically significant for levamisole and 5-FU ($P=0.003$). In sub-set analysis the node-positive group also appeared to benefit from the combination therapy in overall survival. This trial was hypothesis-generating, and therefore required a confirmatory trial. In 1995, Moertel *et al.* (1995b) reported the results of this trial (INT 0035), which confirmed a significant survival benefit and a reduction in recurrence risk after post-operative treatment in patients with stage III disease for levamisole plus 5-FU. Patients with stage III tumours were randomised to one of three arms, identical to those in the original NCCTG trial: (1) surgery alone; (2) surgery plus 12 months of levamisole; (3) surgery plus 12 months of levamisole and 5-FU. The study showed a 15 per cent absolute reduction in the risk of recurrence and a 33 per cent relative reduction in the overall death rate with the combination of surgery plus 5-FU and levamisole. Although there was a trend towards benefit from levamisole alone in the original NCCTG trial, no benefit was seen with levamisole alone in the much larger INT 0035. Notably, neither the NCCTG trial or INT 0035 had a control arm of 5-FU alone, leading to questions as to the exact role of levamisole in this patient population. In INT 0035, patients with stage II disease were randomised to either surgery or 5-FU and levamisole. A trend towards reduction in the rate of disease recurrence in the 5-FU and levamisole arm was observed compared with the surgery-alone group. However, there was no difference in overall survival at a median follow-up duration of seven years. The results in the stage II patients were confounded by both the overall excellent survival with surgery alone, and the small patient population. The overall results of INT 0035, however, established the role of post-operative chemotherapy at least for stage III patients, and the combination of 5-FU and levamisole became the standard therapy for such patients in the USA in 1990 on the basis of an NIH consensus conference. Adoption of adjuvant therapy has gradually become standard practice in most countries, not only on the basis of these trials, but also on the development of other 5-FU-based regimens, which have also demonstrated efficacy in node-positive colon cancer (Table 1.1).

Table 1.1 Five-year disease-free and overall survival rates in recent adjuvant therapy trials for colon cancer

		survival rate (%)	
Adjuvant trial	Regimen	5-yr disease-free	5-yr overall
NSABP C-04	5-FU/levamisole for 1 year	60	69
(stage II & III	5-FU/leucovorin for 8 months	64	74
disease)	5-FU/leucovorin weekly + levamisole for 1 year	64	72
INT 0089	5-FU/levamisole for 1 year	56	63
(high-risk stage	5-FU/leucovorin for 8 months	59	65
II & III disease)	5-FU/leucovorin for 7 months	60	66
	5-FU/leucovorin + levamisole for 7 months	60	67
NCCTG-NCIC	5-FU/levamisole for 6 months	64	63
	5-FU/folinic acid + levamisole for 1 year	66	66
	5-FU/levamisole for 1 year	69	72
	5-FU/leucovorin + levamisole for 6 months	70	75
NSABP C-03	5-FU/leucovorin MOF	73/64*	84/77*

*3-year disease-free and overall-survival rates
5-FU = fluorouracil; MOF = lomustine, vincristine, 5-FU; INT = Intergroup;
NCIC = National Cancer Institute of Canada; NSABP = National Surgical Adjuvant Breast and Bowel Project

A new development in adjuvant treatment has been the use of biochemical modulation of the cytotoxic activity of 5-FU with drugs such as leucovorin (folinic acid). This stabilises the thymidylate synthase complex, maximising and prolonging inhibition (Peeters & Haller 1999), which results in higher degree of tumour response when fluorouracil and leucovorin combinations are compared with bolus fluorouracil used alone (Anonymous 1992).

The International Multicentre Pooled Analysis of Colon Cancer Trials (IMPACT) study analysed pooled data from three studies comparing post-operative fluorouracil and leucovorin to surgery alone: 1,526 patients were randomised, 45 per cent of whom had stage III disease. Patients in the treatment arm had a disease-free survival rate of 62 per cent, compared with 44 per cent in the untreated group after a median follow-up of 37 months (Anonymous 1995).

A direct comparison of standard 5-FU plus levamisole to 5-FU and leucovorin, and also with all three agents together, was performed by the NSABP study (Wolmark *et al.* 1999): 2,151 patients with stage II and III colon cancer were randomised to receive six cycles (12 months of chemotherapy with weekly 5-FU and high-dose leucovorin or one year of either 5-FU and levamisole or the three drugs in combination). The results showed a five-year disease-free survival and overall survival rates of 65 per cent and 74 per cent respectively, for 5-FU and leucovorin, 60 per cent and 70 per cent for the 5-FU and levamisole group, and 64 per cent and 73 per cent for the three-agent combination group. The differences were not statistically significant, but the 5-FU and levamisole group was somewhat inferior to the other two groups. Two conclusions were drawn: a 12-month weekly course of 5-FU and leucovorin was at least as effective as, and possibly superior to, a standard 12-month course of 5-FU and levamisole; levamisole does not add to the survival benefit of 5-FU and leucovorin. Following this, the NCCTG and NCI-Canada compared, in a prospective study, (a) 12 months with six months of treatment and (b) the addition of leucovorin to the standard levamisole regimen. The study showed that 12 months of adjuvant treatment offer no advantage compared with a six-month regimen, and that six months of triple therapy produced a significantly superior survival rate compared with 5-FU and levamisole for the same time period (70 versus 60 per cent) (O'Connell *et al.* 1998).

The second intergroup study (INT-0089) recruited 3,759 patients (20 per cent with high-risk stage II disease) who were randomised to receive standard 5-FU and levamisole for one year, or to seven to eight months of 5-FU and high-dose leucovorin, 5-FU and low-dose leucovorin, or 5-FU and low-dose leucovorin and levamisole (Table 1.2). After a median follow-up of 4.2 years, a marginal survival difference of 1 per cent was demonstrated between the triple therapy arm and the 5-FU/leucovorin arm. On the basis of these trials, seven to eight months of post-operative treatment with 5-FU and leucovorin should represent standard adjuvant treatment for high-risk resected colon cancer patients (Haller *et al.* 1998).

Table 1.2 Treatment arms of Intergroup 0089

Levamisole	50 mg PO every 8 hours for 3 days every 14 days for 1 year	
5-FU	450 mg/m^2 IV bolus for 5 days; on day 29 begin 450 mg/m^2 IV bolus weekly for 48 weeks, for a total treatment of 1 year	
High-dose leucovorin/5-FU	500 mg/m^2 – 2 hr infusion 500 mg/m^2 IV bolus 1 hour after leucovorin infusion started	Repeat weekly x 6, followed by 2-week break period; each 8-week cycle is repeated for a total of 4 courses (24 treatments)
Low dose leucovorin/5-FU	20 mg/m^2 IV bolus 425 mg/m^2 IV bolus	days 1–5; repeat at 4 weeks, 8 weeks then every 5 weeks for a total of 6 courses
Levamisole Leucovorin/5-FU	50 mg PO every 8 hours for 3 days, repeated every 14 days for 6 months 20 mg/m^2 IV bolus 425 mg/m^2 IV bolus	days 1–5; repeat at 4 weeks, 8 weeks, then every 5 weeks for a total of 6 courses
IV = intravenous; PO = oral		

The QUASAR study confirms the conclusion of the INT-0089 study. This study recruited 4,927 patients (28 per cent with stage II disease) who were randomised to receive 5-FU 370mg/m^2 with high dose (175mg) or low dose (25mg) leucovorin and either active or placebo levamisole. The three-year survival was similar with high dose and low dose leucovorin (70.1 per cent versus 71 per cent; p=0.43), as were three-year recurrence rates (36 per cent versus 35.8 per cent; p=0.94). Survival was worse with levamisole than with placebo (69.4 per cent versus 71.5 per cent) at three years (p=0.06), and there were more recurrences with the active drug (37 per cent versus 34.9 per cent) at three years (p=0.16) (QUASAR Collaborative Group 2000).

NSABP study C-05 has compared a standard 5-FU and leucovorin regimen to a similar regimen with the addition of interferon alfa-2a, to explore whether double modulation of fluorouracil might be superior to standard therapy. Patients with stage II and III disease were randomised to six months of 5-FU and leucovorin, with or without interferon alfa-2a. High-grade toxicities were more frequent in the interferon group (22 versus 6 per cent) and no statistically significant difference in survival or disease free survival was observed at four years (Wolmark *et al.* 1998).

Stage II colon cancer

Much of the debate on post-operative adjuvant chemotherapy for stage II patients commenced with the analysis of the Intergroup trial 0035, in which patients with stage II disease showed a reduction in the recurrence rate with post-operative chemotherapy versus surgery alone. The disease-free interval at seven years was 79 per cent for patients randomised to 5-FU and levamisole, compared with 71 per cent of patients in the observation arm. This represents a 32 per cent reduction in the recurrence rate (p=0.10). The overall survival at seven years was 72 per cent for both groups (Moertel *et al.* 1995a). However, the trial was statistically underpowered to assess accurately survival benefits that would be difficult to achieve in a population with such a high cure rate after surgery alone.

A combined analysis of four NSABP adjuvant trials has been conducted, with a total of 1,565 stage II patients. This analysis was aimed to evaluate the magnitude of the benefit of chemotherapy in patients with stage II disease, compared with patients with stage III disease. NSABP C-01, C-02, C-03 and C-04 compared different adjuvant chemotherapy regimens with each other and with no adjuvant treatment (Mamounas *et al.* 1999). In all four studies, the relative overall, disease-free and recurrence-free survival improvement noted for all patients was evident in both stage II and III patients. When the relative efficacy of chemotherapy was examined, there was always an observed reduction in mortality or recurrence or an improvement in disease-free survival, irrespective of stage. In most instances, reduction was as great or greater for stage II as for stage III patients (mortality reduction of 30 per cent for stage II versus 18 per cent for stage III patients). However, the absolute reduction in mortality was much less for the stage II patients, on the basis of their already excellent outcome from surgery alone (Table 1.3).

Table 1.3 Five-year overall survival results in NSABP C-01, C-02, C-03 and C-04, according to stage of disease

Study	All Survival			Stage II Survival			Stage III Survival		
	No.	(%)	P	No.	(%)	P	No.	(%)	P
C-01									
Surgery	375	60	0.07	166	72	0.73	209	50	0.05
MOF	351	67		150	75		201	59	
C-02									
Surgery	343	67	0.08	201	76	0.005	142	56	0.81
PVI	340	74		188	88		152	58	
C-03									
MOF	516	66	0.0008	141	84	0.03	375	59	0.003
5-FU+FA	513	76		149	92		364	70	
C-04									
5-FU+LEV	690	70	0.06	285	81	0.25	405	63	0.21
5-FU+FA	692	75		285	85		407	67	

5-FU = fluorouracil; FA = folinic acid; LEV = levamisole; MOF = lomustine, vincristine, 5-FU; PVI = portal vein infusion

Source: Mamounas *et al.* 1999

Following this analysis, the International Multicentre Pooled Analysis of B2 Colon Cancer Trials was performed (IMPACT B2 1999): 1,016 patients with stage II colon cancer entered into five separate trials were randomised to a 5-FU and leucovorin arm or to an observation arm. The five-year event-free survival was 73 per cent for controls and 76 per cent for the 5-FU and leucovorin arm, and the five-year overall survival was 80 per cent and 82 per cent, respectively. The hazard ratio at five years was 0.83 (90 per cent confidence intervals, 0.72–1.07) for event-free survival and 0.86 (90 per cent confidence intervals, 0.68–1.07) for overall survival. The authors of this report concluded that these data did not support the routine use of 5-FU and leucovorin in all patients with stage II colon cancer.

At this time, there is not universal acceptance of routine adjuvant therapy for stage II colon cancer. Many investigators feel that treatment must be individualised, based on patient preferences and upon possible prognostic markers indicative of poor prognosis. Increasing age and poorly differentiated tumours have been described as significant indicators of poor prognosis in colorectal cancer. Moreover, Moertel *et al.* (1995) noted that the location of a tumour or the presence of perforation or direct organ invasion were independent prognostic factors after multivariate analysis. Markers of nodal positivity in histologic N0 patients have recently been developed. Liefers *et al.* (1998) developed a carcinoembryonic antigen-specific reverse transcriptase polymerase reaction assay, which was able to detect micrometastases in 54 per cent of stage II patients examined in the study. The five-year survival in this group was 50 per cent compared with a five-year survival of 91 per cent in those in whom micrometastases were not detected ($p=0.02$). Tools for the detection of micrometastases may therefore become a useful means of determining a poor-risk sub-set of stage II patients who are likely to benefit from post-operative adjuvant chemotherapy.

Several other parameters have been identified that may function as prognosticators of survival or indicators of response to chemotherapy. Inhibition of thymidylate synthase (TS) has been a major focus for the development of novel therapeutic strategies. It has been suggested that TS overexpression, together with expression of mutant p53, predicts for tumour recurrence and overall survival in stage II colon cancer (Lenz *et al.* 1997). Mutations in p53 alone are associated with a poorer outcome in a number of tumour types, and this may be the case for stage II tumours as well. In addition to the association with fluoropyrimidine resistance, Kitchens *et al.* (1997) reported higher TS expression in colon cancer cell lines, which also expressed a mismatch repair deficient (RER+) phenotype. The Cancer and Leukaemia Group B (1995) report that lack of p27 expression is a predictor of poor prognosis in stage II patients. Loss of chromosome 18q, which results in loss of DCC protein expression, is also related to poorer survival (Jen *et al.* 1994). Some or all of these markers of poor prognosis may predict those patients with high-risk stage II disease, although they all require prospective testing in randomised trials before they are routinely used to select patients for therapy.

Portal vein infusion of 5-FU

Delivery of high doses of chemotherapy to cancer cells may theoretically improve the efficacy of chemotherapy. However, any additional benefit due to high doses of systemic chemotherapy may be outweighed by serious toxic side-effects. Regional chemotherapy, usually with portal vein infusion, may be an alternative approach, since the liver is a major site of disease recurrence. A meta-analysis of ten published trials of 5-FU-based portal vein infusion, including 4,000 patients, identified a modest improvement in overall survival (Anonymous 1997). However, liver metastases were not consistently reduced. The benefit of this approach may be due to a systemic effect, even though it is a regionally administered treatment, since there is not a consistent trend in favour of reduction of liver metastases. Notably, portal vein infusion has often been observed to extend its maximal benefit in patients with stage II disease. Currently, the role of portal vein infusional chemotherapy has not been well defined and remains an experimental approach. On the basis of the possible systemic effect of immediate perioperative intraportal fluorouracil, a US trial of peri-operative systemic fluorouracil is currently under way.

Radiation therapy for extrapelvic colon cancer

The role of adjuvant radiotherapy to reduce the risk of local recurrence in the postoperative setting was evaluated by Willett *et al.* (1993): 173 patients either receiving post-operative radiotherapy (120 patients) or chemotherapy (53 patients) were retrospectively compared with a control group receiving surgery alone. Patients with stage T4, N0 and T4, N1 disease had five-year recurrence-free rates of 93 and 72 per cent respectively, as compared with 69 and 74 per cent in the control groups with equivalent histologic staging. Also, patients with stage III disease showed an improvement in five-year recurrence-free survival with radiotherapy compared with the control group. Patients with T4, N0 disease and perforation or fistula at the tumour site appeared to benefit mostly from adjuvant radiation, with a recurrence-free survival at five years of 91 per cent compared with 43 per cent in the control group. To test whether there was a benefit from radiation in T4, N0 colon cancer in the era of adjuvant therapy with fluorouracil and levamisole, an intergroup trial has been completed in which patients were randomised to the standard chemotherapy regimen, with or without radiation to the tumour bed (Martenson *et al.* 1999). Preliminary results show no benefit from the addition of radiation, with higher toxicity in the combined-modality group. The role of radiation in extrapelvic colon cancer remains controversial.

New drugs and strategies

A number of new drugs and regimens are currently under investigation in the adjuvant setting. An alternative mode of administration of 5-FU, continuous infusion, has been shown to have improved efficacy and decreased haematological toxicity, compared with bolus infusion of 5-FU. A small survival benefit in metastatic colon cancer was also shown with continuous-infusion 5-FU with a survival hazards ratio of 0.88 (p=0.04) (Anonymous 1998). A US intergroup adjuvant trial, comparing the efficacy and toxicity of continuous-infusion fluorouracil to standard bolus fluorouracil and leucovorin has just closed, with preliminary data showing no differences between the treatment approaches (Poplin *et al.* 2000).

Raltitrexed, a quinazoline, is a potent inhibitor of thymidylate synthase. It is polyglutamated and retained within the cells and can be given as a bolus injection every three weeks, a potential advantage over 5-FU therapy. Trials comparing tomudex with 5-FU and leucovorin have shown similar efficacy in response and median survival in metastatic disease (Jackman *et al.* 1995). An adjuvant trial of tomudex compared with standard 5-FU and leucovorin has recently closed prematurely due to high incidence of toxicity reported with tomudex (Ford *et al.* 1999).

Oral fluorinated pyrimidines are currently being incorporated into treatment for metastatic colon cancer. Oral administration allows prolonged exposure to 5-FU, while maintaining a near-constant plasma level of the drug and reducing toxicity due to lower peak concentrations, similar to that seen with continuous intravenous infusions of 5-FU. Uracil-tegafur (UFT) is one of these drugs. Tegafur is 5-FU with a tetrahydrofuran substitution at position 1 of the pyrimidine ring. To date, there is evidence that UFT, given with leucovorin, may be as effective as standard bolus 5-FU and leucovorin in metastatic colon cancer. Its role in the adjuvant setting remains to be determined. In a small Japanese trial of 289 patients who were randomised to UFT (400 mg/day) for two years versus surgery alone, there was a significant difference in disease-free survival (73 versus 62 per cent), but not in overall survival (Nakazato *et al.* 1997). The largest benefit was observed in patients with rectal cancer. The recently completed NSABP C-06 trial was designed to address the role of oral fluoropyrimidines in patients with stages II and III colon cancer, who were randomised to oral UFT and oral leucovorin versus intravenous 5-FU and leucovorin. Capecitabine, S-1 and eniluracil/5-FU are other oral fluoropyrimidine regimens, which may find their own roles in the adjuvant treatment of colon cancer. It is unlikely that any of the oral regimens will be significantly better than standard intravenous regimens, but may have better toxicity profiles and patient acceptance.

Irinotecan (CPT-11) is a topoisomerase I inhibitor with significant single-agent activity in patients with metastatic colorectal cancer refractory to 5-FU or in chemotherapy-naïve patients. Two phase III trials in patients who had already received palliative chemotherapy with a 5-FU regimen, comparing CPT-11 with either best supportive care (Cunningham *et al.* 1998) or a different 5-FU regimen (van Cutsem *et al.* 1998) both showed a survival benefit for CPT-11. Data from randomised trials in advanced-disease patients suggest higher response rates, progression-free survival and overall survival when 5-FU/leucovorin and CPT-11 is compared with 5-FU/leucovorin alone (Saltz *et al.* 1999; Douillard *et al.* 2000). Adjuvant combination chemotherapy trials with CPT-11 plus 5-FU/leucovorin compared with 5-FU/leucovorin are already under way in the USA and Europe.

Oxaliplatin is a diaminocyclohexane platinum derivative. Single-agent oxaliplatin has demonstrated a 10 per cent response rate in patients with 5-FU resistant disease and a 24 per cent response rate when used first line (de Gramont *et al.* 1998). When combined with 5-FU and leucovorin, response rates have been observed as high as 50 per cent (de Gramont *et al.* 1998; Giacchetti *et al.* 2000). Adjuvant trials utilising oxaliplatin-fluorouracil combinations compared to 5-FU/leucovorin have begun in the USA (NSABP C-07) and in Europe (MOSAIC trial).

Monoclonal antibodies

In a randomised, controlled German study of stage III patients, administration of the murine monoclonal antibody 17-1A was compared with no post-operative treatment. A statistically significant reduction in mortality was observed, similar to that observed in trials with chemotherapy alone. Antibody therapy did not reduce local recurrence, but did result in a significant decrease in distant metastases (Riethmüller *et al.* 1998). Toxicity was low and compliance was high in the antibody arm. This trial requires confirmation, as few patients were entered, and there is the possibility of a false positive result. Two large trials of adjuvant chemotherapy, with or without monoclonal antibody 17-1A, have been completed and are awaiting mature analysis.

More recently, an anti-idiotype antibody, designated CeaVac, was developed. This is an integral image of the carcino-embryonic antigen (CEA). Thirty-two patients with resected stages II–IV tumours are currently being followed up, 14 of whom also received 5-FU-based chemotherapy. The remaining only received 2 mg of CeaVac weekly for four weeks and then monthly injections. The preliminary results have demonstrated a potent anti-CEA humoral and cellular immune response consistently generated by CeaVac in all patients. The 5-FU regimens did not affect the immune response. A phase III trial is planned (Foon *et al.* 1999).

Conclusions

Colorectal cancer has remained an important cause of cancer-related mortality. As a result of this, a large number of clinical trials in the adjuvant setting have been performed in an attempt to provide means to improve the outcome in this disease. The role of 5-FU-based therapy in stage III colon cancer was established early on, but the role of adjuvant chemotherapy for stage II disease has remained questionable. Investigations continue towards development of the optimal schedule and duration of chemotherapy, resulting in maximal efficacy with a minimum of toxicity. It appears that a schedule of seven–eight months of 5-FU and leucovorin is as effective as longer regimens and that the addition of levamisole provides no further benefit. Several newer agents such as oral fluoropyrimidines, irinotecan and oxaliplatin, which have demonstrated activity in metastatic disease, are under investigation as potentially effective agents in the adjuvant setting.

References

AbdAlla EE, Blair GE, Jones RA *et al.* (1995). Mechanisms of synergy of levamisole and fluorouracil: Induction of human leucocyte antigen class I in a colorectal cancer cell line. *Journal of the National Cancer Institute* **87**, 489–96.

Anonymous (1992). Modulation of fluorouracil by leucovorin in patients with advances colorectal cancer: evidence in terms of response rate. Advanced Colorectal Cancer Meta-Analysis Project. *Journal of Clinical Oncology* **10**, 896–903.

Anonymous (1995). Efficacy of adjuvant fluorouracil and leucovorin in colon cancer. International Multicentre Pooled Analysis of Colon Cancer Trials (IMPACT). *Lancet* **345**, 939–44.

Anonymous (1997). Portal vein chemotherapy for colorectal cancer: A meta-analysis of 4000 patients in 10 studies. Liver Infusion Meta-Analysis Group. *Journal of the National Cancer Institute* **89**, 497–505.

Anonymous (1998). Efficacy of intravenous continuous infusion of fluorouracil compared with bolus administration in advanced colorectal cancer. Meta-Analysis Group in Cancer. *Journal of Clinical Oncology* **16**, 301–8.

Buyse M, Zeleniuch-Jacquotte A & Chalmers TC (1988). Adjuvant therapy of colorectal cancer: why we still don't know. *Journal of the American Medical Association* **259**, 3571–7.

Cancer and Leukaemia Group B (1995). *Phase III randomised study of adjuvant immunotherapy with monoclonal antibody 17-1A versus no adjuvant therapy following resection for stage II adenocarcinoma of the colon.* Appendix IV.

Cunningham D, Pyrhonen S, James RD *et al.* (1998). Randomised trial of Irinotecan plus supportive care versus supportive care alone after fluorouracil failure for patients with metastatic colorectal cancer. *Lancet* **352**, 1418–8.

De Gramont A, Figer A, Seymour M *et al.* (1998). A randomised trial of leucovorin (LV) and 5 fluorouracil (5FU) with or without oxaliplatin in advanced colorectal cancer (CRC). *Proceedings of the American Society of Clinical Oncology* **17**, 257a, (abstr).

Douillard JY, Cunningham D, Roth AD *et al.* (2000). Irinotecan combined with fluorouracil compared with fluorouracil alone as first line treatment for metastatic colorectal cancer. A multicentre randomised trial. *Lancet* **355**, 1041–7.

Fielding P (1995). Staging systems. In *Cancer of the colon, rectum and anus* (ed. A Cohen & S Winawer), p.207. McGraw Hill, New York, USA.

Foon K, John W, Chakraborty M *et al.* (1999). Clinical and immune responses in resected colon cancer patients treated with anti-idiotype monoclonal antibody vaccine that mimics the carcinoembryonic antigen. *Journal of Clinical Oncology* **17**, 2889.

Ford H & Cunningham D (1999). Correspondence: safety of raltitrexed. *Lancet* **354**, 1824.

Francini G, Petrioli R, Luciano L *et al.* (1994). Leucovorin and 5 fluorouracil as adjuvant chemotherapy in colon cancer. *Gastroenterology* **106**, 899–906.

Giacchetti S, Perpoint B, Zidani R *et al.* (2000). Phase III multicentre randomised trial of oxaliplatin added to chronomodulated fluorouracil. Leucovorin as first-line treatment of metastatic colorectal cancer. *Journal of Clinical Oncology* **18**, 136.

Haller DG, Catalano PJ, Macdonald JS *et al.* (1998). Fluorouracil, leucovorin and levamisole adjuvant therapy for colon cancer. Five year final report of Int-0089. *Proceedings of the American Society of Clinical Oncology* **17**, 256a (abstr).

International Multicentre Pooled Analysis of B2 Colon Cancer Trials Investigators (1999). Efficacy of adjuvant fluorouracil and leucovorin in B2 colon cancer. *Journal of Clinical Oncology* **17**, 1356–63.

Jackman AL & Calvert AH (1995). Folate-based thymidilate synthase inhibitors as anticancer drugs. *Annals of Oncology* **6**, 871–81.

Jen J, Kim H, Piantadosi S *et al.* (1994). Allelic loss of chromosome 18q and prognosis in colorectal cancer. *New England Journal of Medicine* **331**, 213–21.

Kitchens ME & Berger FG (1997). The relationship between mismatch repair defects and expression of thymidylate synthase in fluoropyrimidine-sensitive and –resistant colon tumour cell lines. *Proceedings of the American Society of Clinical Oncology* **38**, 614.

Lenz HJ, Leichman CL, Danenberg KD *et al.* (1995). Thymidylate synthase mRNA level in adenocarcinoma of the stomach: a predictor for primary tumour response and overall survival. *Journal of Clinical Oncology* **14**, 176–82.

Li MC & Ross ST (1976). Chemoprophylaxis for patients with colorectal cancer. Prospective study with five year follow up. *Journal of the American Medical Association* **235**, 2825–8.

Liefers GJ, Cleton-Jansen AM, van de Velde CJH *et al.* (1998). Micrometastases and survival in stage II colon cancer. *New England Journal of Medicine* **339**, 223–8.

Mamounas EP, Weiand S, Wolmark N *et al.* (1999). Comparative efficacy of adjuvant chemotherapy in patients with Dukes' B vs Dukes' C colon cancer: results from four NSABP studies (C-01, C-02, C-03, C-04). *Journal of Clinical Oncology* **17**, 1349.

Martensen J, Willett C, Sargent D *et al.* (1999). A phase III study of adjuvant radiation therapy, 5 fluorouracil and levamisole versus 5 fluorouracil and levamisole in selected patients with resected high risk colon cancer: initial results of INT 0130. *Proceedings of the American Society of Clinical Oncology* **18**, 904.

Merangolo M, Pezzuoli G, Marubini E *et al.* (1989). Adjuvant chemotherapy with fluorouracil and CCNU in colon cancer. Results of a multicentre randomised study. *Tumori* **75**, 269–76.

Moertel CG, Fleming TR, Macdonald JS *et al.* (1995a). Fluorouracil plus levamisole as effective adjuvant therapy after resection of stage III colon carcinoma. *Annals of Internal Medicine* **122**, 321–6.

Moertel CG, Fleming TR, Macdonald JS *et al.* (1995b). Intergroup study of fluorouracil plus levamisole as adjuvant therapy for stage II/Dukes' B2 colon cancer. *Journal of Clinical Oncology* **13**, 2936–43.

Nakazato H, Koike A, Sail S *et al.* (1997). Efficacy of oral UFT as adjuvant chemotherapy to curative resection of colorectal cancer: A prospective randomised clinical trial. *Proceedings of the American Society of Clinical Oncology* **16**, 279a (abstr).

O'Connell MJ, Laurie JA, Kuhn M *et al.* (1998). Prospectively randomised trial of postoperative adjuvant chemotherapy in patients with high risk colon cancer. *Journal of Clinical Oncology* **16**, 295–300.

Panettiere FJ, Goodman PJ, Costanti JJ *et al.* (1988). Adjuvant therapy in large bowel adenocarcinoma: long term results of a Southwest Oncology Group Study. *Journal of Clinical Oncology* **6**, 947–54.

Peeters M & Haller D (1999). Therapy for early stage colorectal cancer. *Oncology* **13**, 307–15.

Pisani P, Parkin DM & Ferlay J (1993). Estimates of worldwide mortality rate from 18 major cancers in 1985: implications for prevention and projections of future burden. *International Journal of Cancer* **55**, 891–903.

Poplin E, Benedetti J, Estes W *et al.* (2000). Phase III randomised trial of bolus 5-FU/leucovorin vs 5-FU continuous infusion levamisole as adjuvant therapy for high-risk colon cancer. *Proceedings of the American Society of Clinical Oncology* 240a.

QUASAR Collaborative Group (2000). Comparison of fluorouracil with additional levamisole, higher dose folinic acid, or both, as adjuvant chemotherapy for colorectal cancer: a randomised trial. *Lancet* **355**, 1588–95.

Riethmuller G, Holz E, Schlimok G *et al.* (1998). Monoclonal antibody therapy for resected Duke's C colorectal cancer: seven year outcome of a multicenter randomised trial. *Journal of Clinical Oncology* **16**, 1788–94.

Saltz LB, Locker PK, Pirotta N *et al.* (1999). Weekly irinotecan, leucovorin and fluorouracil is superior to daily 5 fluorouracil/leucovorin in patients with previously untreated metastatic colorectal cancer. *Proceedings of the American Society of Clinical Oncology* **18**, 898.

van Cutsem E, Bajetta A, Niederle N *et al.* (1998). A phase III multicenter randomised trial comparing CPT-11 to infusional 5FU regimen in patients with advanced colorectal cancer (ACRC) after 5FU failure. *Proceedings of the American Society of Clinical Oncology* **17**, 256a (abstr).

Willett CG, Fung CY, Kaufman DS *et al.* (1993). Postoperative radiation therapy for high risk colon carcinoma. *Journal Clinical Oncology* **11**, 1112–17.

Wolmark N, Fisher B, Rockette H *et al.* (1988). Postoperative adjuvant chemotherapy or BCG for colon cancer. Results from NSABP protocol C-01. *Journal of the National Cancer Institute* **80**, 30–6.

Wolmark N, Bryant J, Smith R *et al.* (1998). Adjuvant 5 fluorouracil and leucovorin with or without interferon alfa-2a in colon carcinoma: National Surgical Adjuvant Breast and Bowel Project Protocol C-05. *Journal of the National Cancer Institute* **90**, 1810–16.

Wolmark N, Rockette H, Mamounas E *et al.* (1999). Clinical trial to assess the relative efficacy of fluorouracil and leucovorin, fluorouracil and levamisole, and fluorouracil, leucovorin and levamisole in patients with Dukes' B and C carcinoma of the colon: results from the National Surgical Adjuvant Breast and Bowel Project C-04. *Journal of Clinical Oncology* **17**, 3533–9.

Chapter 2

Challenging the definition of 'best clinical practice': the impact of new and ongoing studies

Clare A Topham

Introduction

Studies conducted mainly in the USA established a combination of 5-fluorouracil (5-FU) and leucovorin (folinic acid) (LV) as the new standard of care in adjuvant treatment of carcinoma of the colon (Poon *et al.* 1991; Wolmark *et al.* 1993; Erlichman *et al.* 1994; O'Connell *et al.* 1997). In reaction to this the Quasar study was set up in the UK in 1994.

The Quasar study

This was a pragmatic study where the investigators simply had to decide for their patients whether there was either a clear or an uncertain indication for chemotherapy. If there was a clear indication, the patient was randomised among four treatment arms, all containing 5-FU at 370 mg/m^2. Half the arms had high-dose LV, and half low-dose LV. Half the arms had levamisole, and half placebo. Investigators could choose to use a once-weekly schedule for 30 weeks: this was chosen as many oncologists had outside clinics where the only practical way of delivering chemotherapy was once weekly. Alternatively, chemotherapy could be given on a five-day-a-week schedule once a month. If the investigator was uncertain as to the value of chemotherapy, he or she randomised between the four treatment arms or observation only.

The trial was extremely successful, accrued rapidly and by October 1997, had randomised 4,927 patients (Figure 2.1, p.23). There was no difference in survival between levamisole and placebo (Figure 2.2, p.24). There was very little difference in toxicity. Levamisole was associated with more skin rashes (Table 2.1, p.22). Survival on high-dose folinic acid versus low-dose folinic acid showed no difference (Figure 2.3, p.24). There was slightly more toxicity on the high dose folinic acid arm, particularly diarrhoea and stomatitis (Table 2.2, p.22). The comparison between the weekly and monthly schedules was not randomised. Survival between the once-weekly group versus the full weekly schedule showed no difference (Figure 2.4, p.25). Toxicity, however, was very markedly worse with the four-weekly schedule, particularly with stomatitis, diarrhoea and neutropenia (Table 2.3, p.22).

The uncertain randomisation continues, and the trial has been renamed Quasar 1. Patients are randomised between the chemotherapy arm, now consisting of 5-FU 370 mg/m^2, low-dose LV and no levamisole or placebo versus observation (Figure 2.5, p.25) (Gray *et al.* 1999). The target recruitment is 2,500 stage Bs and 1,991 patients have already been randomised. The trial should be completed by the end of year 2000.

The PETACC-1 trial

Tomudex (raltitrexed), the new thymidylate synthase inhibitor, has been shown in several trials in advanced disease to have equivalent activity to 5-FU and LV (Cunningham *et al.* 1995, 1996; Zalcberg *et al.* 1996; Pazdur *et al.* 1997; Cocconi *et al.* 1998). It has the advantage of ease of administration, requiring a 15-minute infusion once every three weeks. It was being tested in the adjuvant situation in Europe in the PETACC-1 trial: raltitrexed at a dose of 3 mg/m^2 given three-weekly was compared with the MAYO regimen (Figure 2.6, p.26). The trial was terminated due to toxicity.

Monoclonal antibody treatment

An alternative approach to adjuvant chemotherapy is to use antibody treatment. In the Riethmuller *et al.* study (1998), 189 patients with Dukes' C colon and rectal carcinoma were randomised from six centres in Germany, between five courses of panorex – monoclonal antibody 17-1A – post-surgery, against observation only. Results at seven years showed a statistically significant improvement in recurrence-free survival for panorex (Figure 2.7, p.26), and a statistically significant improvement in overall survival (Figure 2.8, p.27).

This study provided the basis for the monoclonal antibody 17-1A study. Patients with curatively resected Dukes' C carcinoma of the colon were randomised among monoclonal antibody 17-1A alone, 5-FU and LV on the MAYO regimen alone versus monoclonal antibody 17-1A and 5-FU/LV together (Figure 2.9, p.27).

The study closed in March1999, having randomised 2,725 patients worldwide. Results will be reported in late 2000.

5-FU infusion versus 5-FU bolus

The meta-analysis of 5-FU infusion versus 5-FU bolus in advanced disease showed an improved response rate for 5-FU infusion (Figure 2.10, p.28) (Anonymous 1998). The response rate for continuous infusion of 5-FU was 22 versus 14 per cent for bolus 5-FU. There was less haematological toxicity with continuous 5-FU, but more hand-foot syndrome. A study currently running in Europe, PETACC-2, tests 5-FU/LV bolus on the MAYO regimen versus the French LV5-FU2 schedule versus the German and Spanish regimens (Figure 2.11, p.29).

New cytotoxic agents

Oxaliplatin

Studies with oxaliplatin, irinotecan and capecitabine show promise in advanced disease. Oxaliplatin is a platinum derivative in which the platinum atom is complexed with a 1, 2 diaminocyclohexane (DACH) and with an oxalate ligand as a leaving group (Bleiberg *et al.* 1999; Figer *et al.* 1999; Zori Comba *et al.* 1999). A first-line, phase III study in advanced colorectal carcinoma, comparing LV5-FU2 with LV5-FU2 plus oxaliplatin (Figure 2.12, p.30), reported at ASCO, showed improvement, in progression-free survival for LV5-FU2 plus oxaliplatin (Figure 2.13, p.30), with no difference in overall survival (Figure 2.14, p.31), but there was crossover on the study. The response rate of oxaliplatin plus LV5-FU2 was 50 per cent compared with 21.9 per cent for the LV5-FU2 arm alone. The progression-free survival for the combination was 8.2 versus 6 months. Side-effects were acceptable, being mainly neuropathy, associated with oxaliplatin (De Gramont *et al.* 1999).

These promising results led to the design of the MOSAIC study, in which histologically proven Dukes' B and C patients, with the inferior pole of the tumour above the peritoneal reflection, were randomised between 5-FU, LV2 with or without oxaliplatin. This study, opened in October 1998, is accruing rapidly and aims to randomise 1,500 patients in two years (Figures 2.15, p.31 and 2.16, p.32). It is extremely important that patients randomised on an adjuvant study should not develop long-term neurotoxicity, so there is a stringent dose modification schedule in the study for development of neurotoxicity (Table 2.4, p.23).

Irinotecan

Irinotecan is a topoisomerase 1 inhibitor and, added to 5-FU/LV in advanced disease, has been shown to increase the efficacy of 5-FU and LV (Kalbakis *et al.* 1999; Maiello *et al.* 1999; Saltz *et al.* 1999). A study reported by Douillard *et al.* (2000) at ASCO compared FU5 LV2 plus or minus irinotecan. The time to progression was 6.7 months for irinotecan plus 5-FU/LV, compared with 4.4 months, and there was an overall survival for the irinotecan arm of 16.8 months, compared with 14 months for the 5-FU/LV arm (Figure 2.17, p.32).

This study provides the basis for the new irinotecan adjuvant study for Dukes' B and C adenocarcinoma of the colon or higher rectum. Patients will be randomised to irinotecan plus either the AIO regimen or the LV5-FU2 regimen, versus the AIO regimen or LV5-FU2 regimen alone. It is planned to accrue 1,800 patients with Dukes' C colon cancer over three years, at which time it is expected there will be 630 Dukes' B patients randomised (Figures 2.18, p.33 and 2.19, p.34).

New oral 5-FU agents

Finally, there are now new oral 5-FU agents, such as capecitabine, which have been shown in advanced-disease studies to have equivalent response rates to 5-FU/LV (Cox *et al.* 1999; Twelves *et al.* 1999). Capecitabine is an oral tumour-selective fluoropyrimidine with preferential conversion to 5-FU at the tumour site. It exploits the higher levels of thymidine phosphorylase found in tumour tissues compared to normal tissues. It has similar side-effects to 5-FU (e.g. diarrhoea, nausea and vomiting, hand-foot syndrome, fatigue, stomatitis and conjunctivitis), and is currently being tested in the X-ACT study, where surgically resected Dukes' C carcinomas of the colon are randomised between capecitabine versus bolus 5-FU/LV on the MAYO regimen (Figures 2.20, p.34 and 2.21, p.35).

The proposed new Quasar 2 study, planned to start in the UK in year 2000, is a two-by-two factorial design, comparing capecitabine with bolus 5-FU/ LV plus or minus irinotecan (Figure 2.22, p.35).

Conclusion

If capecitabine shows equivalence to 5-FU/LV and if the new agents show superiority in combination with 5-FU/LV in these adjuvant studies, there are many exciting possibilities for simplified or more effective regimens for patients in the future, leading to a whole new standard of care.

References

Anonymous (1998). Efficacy of intravenous continuous infusion of fluorouracil compared with bolus administration in advanced colorectal cancer. The Meta-Analysis Group in Cancer. *Journal of Clinical Oncology* **16**, 301–8

Bleiburg H, Brienza S, Gerard B, Di Leo A, Hendlisz A, Van Deale D, Cornez N, Geurs F, Duriau D & Bertaux B (1999). Oxaliplatin combined with a high dose, 24-hour continuous 5-FU infusion and folinic acid based regimen in patients (pts) with advanced colorectal cancer (CRC). *Proceedings of the American Society of Clinical Oncology* **18**, 925.

Cocconi G, Cunningham D, Van Custem E, Francois E, Gustavsson B, Van Hazel G, Kerr D, Possinger K & Hietschold SM on behalf of the 'Tomudex' Colorectal Cancer Study Group (1998). Open, randomised, multi-centre trial of Raltitrexed versus Fluorouracil plus high dose Leucovorin in patients with advanced colorectal cancer. *Journal of Clinical Oncology* **16**, 2943–52.

Cox JV, Pazdur R, Thibault A, Maroun J, Weaver C, Jahn MW, Harrison E & Griffin T (1999). *Proceedings of the American Society of Clinical Oncology* **18**, 1016.

Cunningham G, Zalcberg J, Rath U, Olver I, Van Cutsem E, Svensson C, Seitz JF, Harper P, Kerr D, Perez-Manga G, Azab M, Seymour L, Lowery K and the Tomudex Colorectal Cancer Study Group (1995). Tomudex (ZD1694): results of a randomised trial in advanced colorectal cancer demonstrate efficacy and reduced mucositis and leucopenia. *European Journal of Cancer* **31** A, 1945–54.

Cunningham G, Zalcberg JR, Rath U, Oliver I, Van Cutsem E, Svensson C, Seitz JF, Harper P, Kerr D, Perez-Manga G and the Tomudex Colorectal Cancer Study Group (1996). Final results of a randomised trial comparing 'Tomudex' (raltitrexed) with 5-fluorouracil plus leucovorin in advanced colorectal cancer. *Annals of Oncology* **7**, 961–5.

De Gramont A, Maindrault-Goebel F, Louvet C, Andre T, Carola E, Gilles-Amar V, Mabro M, Izrael V & Krulik M (1999). Evaluation of oxaliplatin dose-intensity with the bimonthly 48h leucovorin (LV) and 5-fluorouracil (5FU) regimens (FOLFOX) in pretreated metastatic colorectal cancer. *Proceedings of the American Society of Clinical Oncology* **18**, 1018.

Douillard JY, Cunningham D, Roth AD, Germa JR, James RD, Karasek P, Jandik P, Iveson T, Carmichael J, Gruia G, Dembak M, Sibaud D & Rougier P (2000). Irinotecan combined with fluorouracil compared with fluorouracil alone as first line treatment for metastatic colorectal cancer. A multicentre randomised trial. *Lancet* **355**, 1041–7.

Erlichman C, Marsoni S, Seitz JF *et al.* (1994). Event-free and overall survival is increased by FU/FA in resected B and C colon cancer: a prospective pooled analysis of 3 randomized trials (RCTS). *Proceedings of the American Society of Clinical Oncology* **13**, 194.

Figer A, Louvet C, Homerin M, Hmissi A, Seymour M, Cassidy J & Boni C (1999). Analysis of prognostic factors of overall survival (OS) in the randomized trial of bimonthly leucovorin and 5-fluorouracil regimen (LV5FU2) with or without oxaliplatin (OXA) in advanced colorectal cancer (ACC). *Proceedings of the American Society of Clinical Oncology* **18**, 918.

Gray R *et al.* (1999). Quasar: a UKCCCR study of adjuvant chemotherapy (CT) for colorectal cancer. *ECCO* September.

Kalbakis K, Kandylis N, Stavrakakis J, Varthalitis J, Giannakakis Th, Athanasiadis A, Potamianou A, Demiri M, Kouroussis Ch, Mavroudis D, Kakolyris S, Sarra E, Hatzidaki D, Samonis G & Georgoulias V (1999). First line chemotherapy with 5-fluorouracil (5-FU), leucovorin (LV) and irinotecan (CPT-11) in advanced colorectal cancer (CRC): a multicenter phase II study. *Proceedings of the American Society of Clinical Oncology* **18**, 989.

Maiello, E, Giuliani F, Gebbia V, Cigolari S, Fortunato S, Paoletti G, Borsellino N, Gebbia N, Lopez M & Colucci G (1999). Bi-monthly folinic acid (FA) and 5-fluorouracil (FU) bolus and continuous infusion alone or with irinotecan (CPT-11) for advanced colorectal cancer (ACC): preliminary results of a phase II randomized trial of the Southern Italy Oncology Group. *Proceedings of the American Society of Clinical Oncology* **18**, 929.

O'Connell M, Malliard J, Kahn MJ *et al.* (1993). Control trial of fluorouracil and low-dose leucovorin given for six months as post-operative adjuvant therapy for colon cancer. *Journal of Clinical Oncology* **11**, 1879–87.

Pazdur R & Vincent M (1997). Raltitrexed (Tomudex) versus 5-fluorouracil and leucovorin (5FU+LV) in patients with advanced colorectal cancer (ACC): results of a randomized, multicenter, North American trial. *Proceedings of the American Society of Clinical Oncology* **16**, 801.

Poon MA, O'Connell MJ, Wieand HS *et al.* (1991). Biochemical modulation of fluorouracil with leucovorin: confirmatory evidence of improved therapeutic efficacy in advanced colorectal cancer. *Journal of Clinical Oncology* **9**, 1967–72.

Riethmuller G, Holz E, Schlimok G, Schmiegel W, Raab R, Hoffken K, Gruber R, Funke I, Pichlmaier H, Hirche H, Buggisch P, Witte J & Pichlmayr R (1998). Monoclonal antibody therapy for resected Dukes' C colorectal cancer: seven-year outcome of a multicenter randomized trial. *Journal of Clinical Oncology* **16**, 1788–94.

Saltz LB, Locker PK, Pirotta N, Elfring GL & Miller LL (1999). Weekly irinotecan (CPT-11), leucovorin (LV), and fluorouracil (FU) is superior to daily x5LV/FU in patients (PTS) with previously untreated metastatic colorectal cancer (CRC). *Proceedings of the American Society of Clinical Oncology* **18**, 898.

Twelves C, Harper P, Van Custem E, Thibault A, Shelygin YA, Burger HU, Allman D & Osterwalder B (1999). *Proceedings of the American Society of Clinical Oncology* **18**, 1010.

Wolmark N, Rockette H, Fisher B *et al.* (1993). The benefit of leucovorin-modulated fluorouracil as postoperative adjuvant therapy for primary colon cancer: results from national surgical adjuvant breast and bowel project protocol C-03. *Journal of Clinical Oncology* **11**, 1879–87.

Zalcberg JR, Cunningham D, Van Cutsem E, Francois E, Schornagel J, Adenis A, Green M, Iveson A, Azab M & Seymour I (1996). ZD 1694: a novel thimidylate synthase inhibitor with substantial activity in the treatment of patients with advanced colorectal cancer. *Journal of Clinical Oncology* **14**, 716–21.

Zori Comba A, Blajman C, Richardet E, Vilanova M, Coppola F, Van Kooten M, Rodger J, Giglio R, Balbiani L, Perazzo F, Montiel M, Chacon M, Pujol E, Mickiwicz E, Cazap G, Recondo M, Kotliar P, Nesis M, Reale F, Lastiri A & Schmilovich (1999). Bimonthly oxaliplatin (L-OHP) with (A) or without (B) fluorouracil (FU) and leucovorin (FA): proven evidence of synergism in a phase II: randomised trial. *Proceedings of the American Society of Clinical Oncology* **18**, 953.

Appendix: Figures and tables

Table 2.1 Toxicity events reported

	Levamisole Events	Placebo Events	Odds ratio (95% CI)
Nausea & Vomiting	173	143	1.23 (0.98–1.55)
Stomatitis	181	191	0.95 (0.77–1.17)
Diarrhoea	337	356	0.93 (0.80–1.10)
Neutropenia	109	117	0.93 (0.71–1.22)

$p > 0.05$ for all comparisons

Table 2.2 Toxicity events reported

	High dose FA Events	Low dose FA Events	Odds ratio (95% CI)
Nausea & Vomiting	169	150	1.14 (0.91–1.43)
Stomatitis	216	158	1.40* (1.13–1.74)
Diarrhoea	362	338	1.08 (0.92–1.27)
Neutropenia	111	116	0.95 (0.73–1.25)

$p > 0.05$ for all comparisons except *$p = 0.002$

Table 2.3 Toxicity events reported, schedule comparison, non-randomised.

	Weekly schedule Events	4-weekly schedule Events
Nausea & Vomiting	130	148
Stomatitis	31	291
Diarrhoea	221	378
Any haematological	19	135

Table 2.4 Dose modification of oxaliplatin (mg/m^2/course)

Duration/Type of toxicity	≤ 7 days	> 7 days < 14 days	Persistent in between courses
Cold related dysesthesia	None	None	None
Paresthesia without pain	None	None	STOP until recovery Then restart at 75 mg/m^2
Paresthesia with pain	None	Reduction:75*	STOP
Paresthesia with functional impairment	None	Reduction:75*	STOP

Figure 2.1 Quasar

- Apparently curative surgery for colorectal cancer
- ? Role for 6 months adjuvant chemotherapy

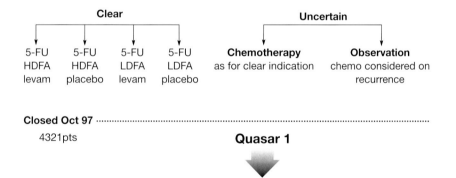

Clear				**Uncertain**	
5-FU HDFA levam	5-FU HDFA placebo	5-FU LDFA levam	5-FU LDFA placebo	**Chemotherapy** as for clear indication	**Observation** chemo considered on recurrence

Closed Oct 97 ··

4321pts

Quasar 1

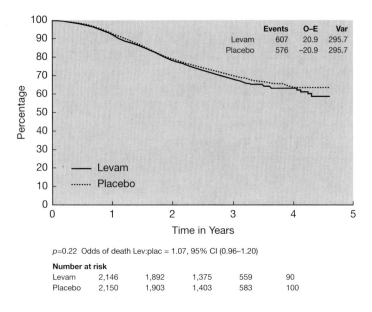

Figure 2.2 Survival, clear indication, levamisole versus placebo

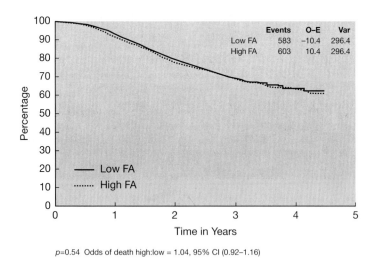

p=0.54 Odds of death high:low = 1.04, 95% CI (0.92–1.16)

Figure 2.3 Survival, clear indication, high- versus low-dose FA

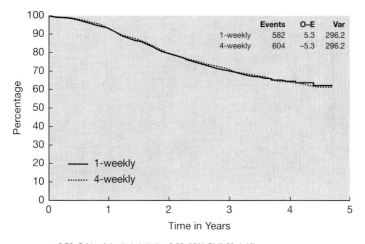

p=0.76 Odds of death 4wk:1wk = 0.98, 95% CI (0.88–1.10)

Figure 2.4 Survival, clear indication, 1-weekly versus 4-weekly schedule

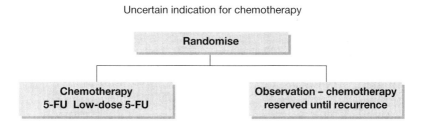

Figure 2.5 Quasar 1 trial design

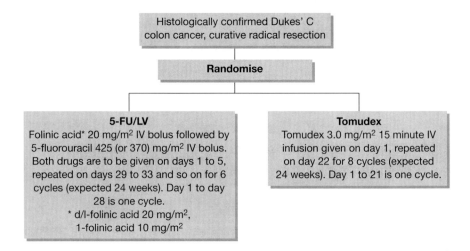

Figure 2.6 PETACC-1 trial design

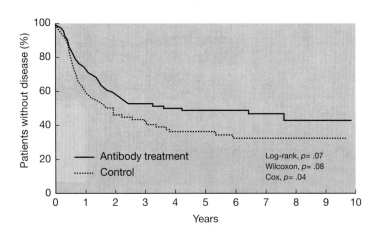

Figure 2.7 Recurrence-free survival after seven years of follow-up

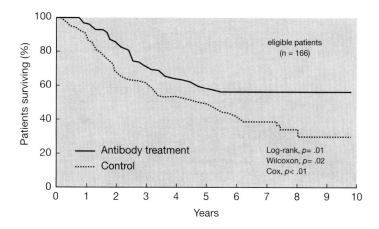

Figure 2.8 Overall survival of patients after seven years of follow-up

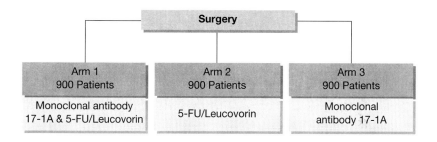

Figure 2.9 Monoclonal antibody 17-1A study design

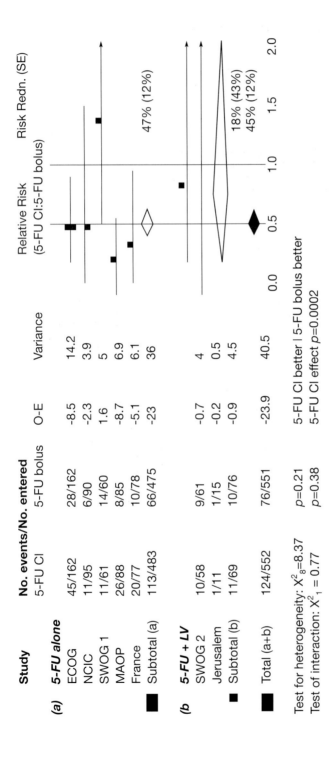

Study	No. events/No. entered		O-E	Variance	Relative Risk (5-FU CI:5-FU bolus)	Risk Redn. (SE)
	5-FU CI	5-FU bolus				
(a) 5-FU alone						
ECOG	45/162	28/162	-8.5	14.2		
NCIC	11/95	6/90	-2.3	3.9		
SWOG 1	11/61	14/60	1.6	5		
MAOP	26/88	8/85	-8.7	6.9		
France	20/77	10/78	-5.1	6.1		
Subtotal (a)	113/483	66/475	-23	36		47% (12%)
(b 5-FU + LV						
SWOG 2	10/58	9/61	-0.7	4		
Jerusalem	1/11	1/15	-0.2	0.5		
Subtotal (b)	11/69	10/76	-0.9	4.5		18% (43%)
Total (a+b)	124/552	76/551	-23.9	40.5		45% (12%)

Test for heterogeneity: $X^2_8=8.37$ $p=0.21$

Test of interaction: $X^2_1 = 0.77$ $p=0.38$

5-FU CI better | 5-FU bolus better

5-FU CI effect $p=0.0002$

Figure 2.10 Tumour response OR in individual trials and overall. O, Observed; E, expected; Risk Redn, reduction in the odds of not achieving a tumour response. (Test for treatment effect, $p=.0002$)

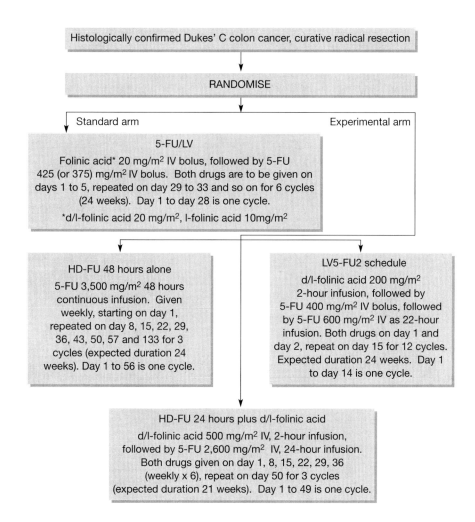

Figure 2.11 PETACC-2 trial design

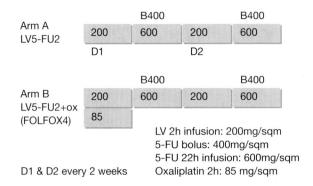

Figure 2.12 Phase III study of 5-FU/leucovorin + oxaliplatin

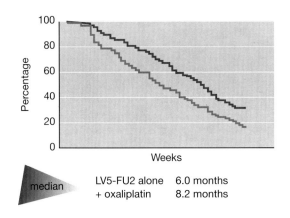

Figure 2.13 Progression-free survival

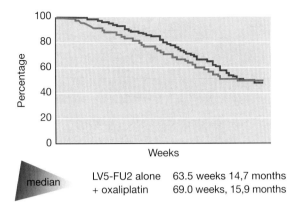

LV5-FU2 alone   63.5 weeks 14,7 months
+ oxaliplatin   69.0 weeks, 15,9 months

Figure 2.14 Overall survival

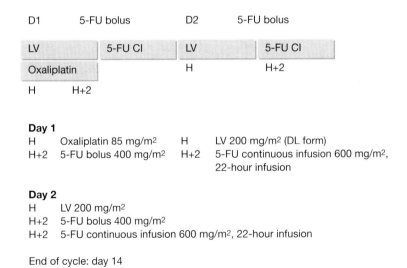

Day 1

| H | Oxaliplatin 85 mg/m^2 | H | LV 200 mg/m^2 (DL form) |
| H+2 | 5-FU bolus 400 mg/m^2 | H+2 | 5-FU continuous infusion 600 mg/m^2, 22-hour infusion |

Day 2

H   LV 200 mg/m^2
H+2 5-FU bolus 400 mg/m^2
H+2 5-FU continuous infusion 600 mg/m^2, 22-hour infusion

End of cycle: day 14

Figure 2.15 Arm A: LV5-FU2 + oxaliplatin

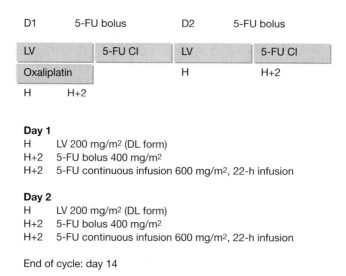

Day 1

H	LV 200 mg/m² (DL form)
H+2	5-FU bolus 400 mg/m²
H+2	5-FU continuous infusion 600 mg/m², 22-h infusion

Day 2

H	LV 200 mg/m² (DL form)
H+2	5-FU bolus 400 mg/m²
H+2	5-FU continuous infusion 600 mg/m², 22-h infusion

End of cycle: day 14

Figure 2.16 Arm B: LV5-FU2

	Irino + 5-FU/FA	5-FU/FA	p-value
No. of eligible patients	198	187	$p<0.001$
OPR (evaluable patients)	41%	23%	$p<0.001$
Duration of response and stabilisation	8.6 mths	6.2 mths	$p<0.001$
TTP	6.7 mths	4.4 mths	$p=0.001$
Time to treatment failure	5.3 mths	3.8 mths	$p=0.001$
Probability of survival at 12 mths	69%	59%	$p=0.03$
Overall survival	16.8 mths	14 mths	$p=0.03$

Figure 2.17 Efficacy results (full analysis)

A1. HD-FU 24 hours plus folinic acid, every week (AIO-schedule)

Irinotecan	80 mg/m^2 as a 60-minute infusion given on days 1, 8, 15, 22, 29, 36 (weekly x 6)

*Folinic acid**	500 mg/m^2 IV, 2-hour infusion, followed by
5-FU	2,000 mg/m^2 IV, 24-hour infusion, both drugs given on days 1, 8, 15, 22, 29, 36 (weekly x 6)

This sequence is repeated on day 50.

Day 1–50 is one cycle.

A2. Bolus and infusional high-dose 5-FU + folinic acid every 2 weeks (LV5-FU2 regimen)

On day 1:

Irinotecan	180 mg/m^2 as a 60-minute infusion

On days 1 and 2:

*Folinic acid**	200 mg/m^2 as a 2-hour infusion followed by
5-FU	5-FU 400 mg/m^2 as a bolus and then 5-FU 600 mg/m^2 as a 22-hour continuous infusion

Day 1 is repeated on day 15.

Day 1–15 is one cycle.
*or half dose, 250 mg/m^2 or 100 mg/m^2 respectively in case of use of L-folinic acid.

Figure 2.18 Group A: Irinotecan + high-dose infusional 5-FU/folinic acid (either AIO regimen or LV5-FU2 regimen)

B1. AIO regimen: the dose of 5-FU is 2,600 mg/m² compared to 2,000 mg/m² in group A1

Folinic acid*   500 mg/m² IV, 2-hour infusion, followed by 5-FU 2,600mg/m² IV, 24-hour infusion, both drugs given on days 1, 8, 15, 22, 29, 36 (weekly x 6)

Day 1 is repeated on day 50   Day 1–50 is one cycle
*or half dose, 250 mg/m² or 100mg/m² respectively in case of use of L-folinic acid

B2. LV5-FU2 regimen: the doses of 5-FU are the same as the doses used in the combination group

On day 1 and day 2

Folinic acid*   200 mg/m² as a 2-hour infusion, followed by 5-FU 400 mg/m² as a bolus and then 5-FU 600 mg/m² as a 22-hour continuous infusion

Day 1 is repeated on day 15   Day 1–15 is one cycle
*or half dose, 250 mg/m² or 100 mg/m² respectively in case of use of L-folinic acid

Duration of treatment: 6 months for both groups

Concomitant medications

In group A, a pre-medication is mandatory, consisting of anti-emetics. Prophylactic pre-medication with atropine is allowed from the first cycle in group A, provided the absence of contra-indications was checked.

Figure 2.19 Group B: high-dose infusional 5-FU alone

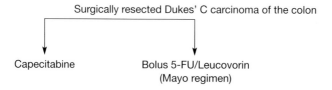

Surgically resected Dukes' C carcinoma of the colon

Capecitabine   Bolus 5-FU/Leucovorin
(Mayo regimen)

Figure 2.20 X-Act study

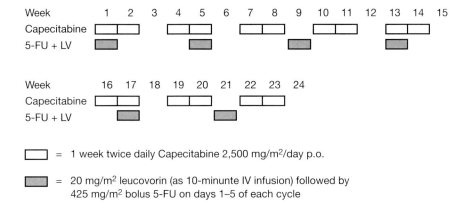

Week	1	2	3	4	5	6	7	8	9	10	11	12	13	14	15

Capecitabine
5-FU + LV

Week	16	17	18	19	20	21	22	23	24

Capecitabine
5-FU + LV

☐ = 1 week twice daily Capecitabine 2,500 mg/m^2/day p.o.

▨ = 20 mg/m^2 leucovorin (as 10-minunte IV infusion) followed by 425 mg/m^2 bolus 5-FU on days 1–5 of each cycle

Figure 2.21 X-Act study design

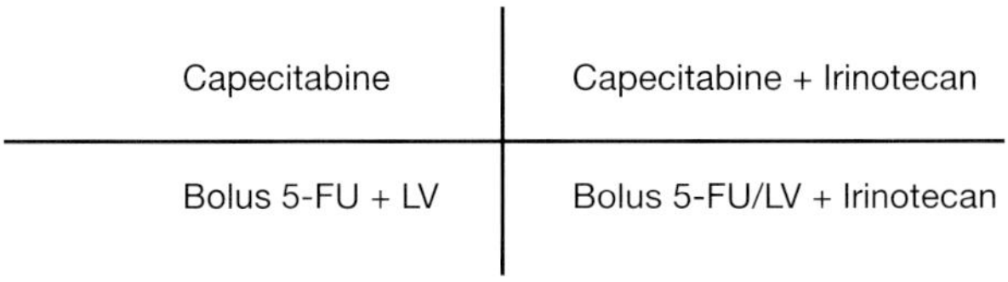

Capecitabine	Capecitabine + Irinotecan
Bolus 5-FU + LV	Bolus 5-FU/LV + Irinotecan

Figure 2.22 Quasar 2

Chapter 3

Is adjuvant intrahepatic infusion defunct?

Roger James

Introduction

Colorectal cancer (CRC) is the third most important cause of cancer-related mortality, causing around 0.5 million deaths annually worldwide. The liver is the most important site for metastases, probably as a result of portal venous dissemination. Adjuvant systemic chemotherapy for node-positive (Dukes' C) colorectal cancer, delivered over six months as for breast cancer, is now accepted to result in a small, but important survival advantage (Moertel *et al.* 1995). Modern randomised clinical trials of adjuvant chemotherapy in CRC distinguish node-positive from node-negative patients. Consensus statements suggest it is now unethical to include a no-treatment arm for node-positive patients.

The median age for colorectal cancer is much higher than for breast cancer and more patients, with an increased prevalence of medical co-morbidity, are unable to tolerate conventional bolus chemotherapy. Portal vein infusion (PVI) of cytotoxic drugs has been proposed as a useful alternative strategy, particularly as the portal venous system is accessible during conventional colonic resections. Portal cannulation, once learned, adds only 15 minutes to the operation.

There are a number of reasons for testing the proposition that adjuvant PVI might reduce deaths from colorectal cancer. Cytotoxic drugs administered systemically produce relatively low doses in the liver compared with intrahepatic infusion (Goldberg *et al.* 1988). Furthermore, randomised advanced disease studies report response rates following arterial infusion of 5-fluorouracil (5-FU) which exceed those from equivalent systemic infusion (Taylor *et al.* 1985).

Early, non-randomised studies using thiotepa and mechlorethamine (Morales *et al.* 1957; Holden & Dixon 1962) produced unacceptable toxicity, and in recent years 5-FU or 5-FU analogues have been the agents of choice. Most published studies of PVI have used a seven-day infusion of 5-FU delivered in the immediate post-operative period, a technique clearly more cost-effective than six months of adjuvant intravenous bolus chemotherapy, and some have reported survival advantage similar to those from intravenous bolus studies. The mechanism of such equi-effectiveness is unclear, but may be due to physiological differences in the post-operative period rather than a direct effect on the liver. One study of PVI reported a reduction in extrahepatic recurrences, but no reduction in hepatic recurrences (Wolmark *et al.* 1990).

A strategy to prevent line thrombosis in most published trials is the daily administration of PVI heparin in saline. Most studies use an infusion of 1 gram of 5-FU plus 5,000 units of heparin in 1 litre of 5 per cent dextrose infused at a constant rate over each 24-hour period, giving a total of 7 grams of 5-FU over seven days. It has been argued that heparin might be responsible for any reduction in metastases but three-arm studies (Wereldsma et al. 1990; Fielding et al. 1992) appear to refute this. Haematological and biochemical monitoring should be performed at least on alternate days during PVI and immediately prior to discharge. 5-FU is usually stopped if WBC <3.5 x 109/l or platelets <100 x 10^9/l (resuming if blood counts recovered), and if stomatitis, severe diarrhoea or any severe post-operative complication occur.

Serious post-operative complications do not appear to be increased as a result of PVI. Data from the largest randomised trial, AXIS, showed that post-operative deaths (i.e. within 30 days) occurred in 2.7 per cent of those allocated 5-FU and in 3.6 per cent of those allocated 5-FU – a difference which is not statistically significant (P=0.1).

In AXIS there appeared to be a statistically significantly higher number of minor, non-life-threatening complications in the PVI group. The open-ended, subjective question asked of surgeons on complications made over-reporting in one arm a possibility. The only specific complications which were statistically significant ($\chi^2 \, p$ value <0.01) were of anastomotic nature (leakage, dehiscence), and occurred in 2.1 per cent of those allocated no 5-FU and 3.6 per cent of those allocated 5-FU (James 1999).

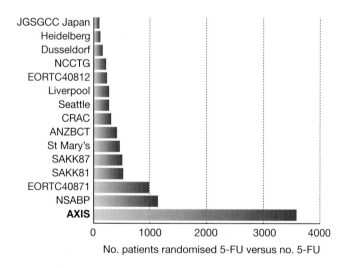

Figure 3.1 Published trials of adjuvant PVI in colorectal cancer

Early trials (1980–1990)

Early trials of PVI included both rectal and colonic cancers, although it is now recognised that the two diseases should be considered separately. Compared with colon cancer, rectal cancer is more likely to recur locally, outcome is more dependent on surgical technique and patients are more likely to benefit from peri-operative pelvic radiotherapy (XRT). Recent studies suggest that survival benefit following adjuvant systemic chemotherapy is less likely with rectal than with colon cancer.

The first randomised trial to test adjuvant PVI of 5-FU was carried out by Taylor *et al.* (1985), who reported highly encouraging results. The succeeding 15 years saw a succession of similar trials with conflicting results, powered to detect large survival differences similar to that reported in the original study.

The first Swiss SAKK group used continuous 5-FU infusion (500 mg/m^2 daily for seven days) with mitomycin C (10 mg/m^2) on day 1. Only 83 per cent of the 236 patients complied with full protocol doses. At median follow up of eight years there was a reduction in the risk of death of 26 per cent, compared with no difference at 42 months (Metzger *et al.* 1987; SAKK 1995).

A joint NCCTG/Mayo clinic study which randomised 219 patients to either surgery plus 5-FU PVI or surgery alone, showed no differences in the frequency of liver metastases at 66 months (Beart *et al.* 1990). The much larger NSABP trial enrolled 1,158 patients, but excluded 257 from analysis because of unresectable disease, while survival data were available on only 33 per cent of patients at four years. However, in this remaining group, the collaborators reported a disease-free survival advantage (Wolmark *et al.* 1990). A trial of 302 patients randomised between 5-FU, heparin PVI versus heparin PVI reported an improvement in survival, with a reduction in liver metastases in the treatment arm which emerged with increasing significance from three to five years (Fielding *et al.* 1992).

More recent trials (1990–2000)

A meta-analysis in 1991 suggested a reduction of about one-third in the risk of death for patients allocated PVI of 5-FU (Gray *et al.* 1991). A subsequent meta-analysis in 1997 of 4,000 patients in ten trials, suggested a projected 10–15 per cent reduction in the odds of death, corresponding to an absolute five-year survival improvement of about 5 per cent, with an estimated reduction in liver metastases by 25 per cent (Liver Infusion Meta-Analysis Group 1997). However, two recent trials (SAKK 81 and EORTC 40871) have questioned this.

The second Swiss SAKK 81 trial randomised 769 patients with colon or rectal cancer among three arms: 5-FU PVI, 5-FU venous infusion and control. At median follow-up of five years, there were no significant differences in disease-free survival. However, the trial was unusual by including an excess (65 per cent) of node-negative patients, which would reduce the prevalence of cancer events at follow-up compared with other published trials (Laffer *et al.* 1998).

The EORTC 40871 trial, which randomised 1,235 patients between 5-FU PVI (500 mg/m^2) and control, showed no significant differences at five years in survival or incidence of liver metastases (Rougier et al. 1998).

The Adjuvant X-Ray Infusion Study (AXIS), launched in November 1989 by the United Kingdom Coordinating Committee for Cancer Research (UKCCCR), is by far the largest study of 5-FU PVI, although a Chinese trial is in progress, with an accrual target of 8,000 patients. Preliminary data from AXIS were presented at ASCO 1999 (James 1999). The trial was designed to be large enough to confirm or refute any survival advantage to adjuvant PVI and peri-operative pelvic XRT in patients with potentially curable colorectal cancer. The trial was closed in 1997 with 3,681 patients randomised. AXIS was the first PVI trial to formalise the distinction between rectal and colon cancer and investigate the interaction between pelvic XRT and PVI. A total of 3,583 patients were randomised with respect to 5-FU. Patient age ranged from 19 to 92, with a median of 68; 57 per cent had colon tumours and 59 per cent were male.

AXIS used the uncertainty principle for randomisation. The only eligibility criteria were that the patient had suspected colorectal cancer and was fit to receive 5-FU, and that the responsible surgeon was uncertain as to whether intra-portal chemotherapy was indicated. In addition, rectal cancer patients could be randomised with respect to both 5-FU and XRT (this was encouraged) or XRT alone. The choice of pre- or post-operative XRT was made on a per-patient basis before randomisation. Both randomisations took place simultaneously and thus pre-operatively, with the exception of patients randomised with respect to post-operative XRT alone, for whom post-operative randomisation was possible. Both colon and rectal cancer patients could be randomised with respect to 5-FU. Where this was the only randomisation, it was to take place as close as possible to the time of surgery, and preferably intra-operatively. A small number of patients in AXIS were randomised with known metastases – this was permitted by the protocol and occurred mainly in the early years of the trial.

In AXIS patients with rectal cancer could be randomised to receive pre-operative pelvic XRT or no XRT. A variety of XRT schedules were permitted, the intention being that radical XRT should be delivered, with appropriate shielding, while taking into account local variations in XRT fractionation that had arisen from local experience, logistic or economic considerations. For pre-operative XRT, the recommended schedules were 25 Gy in four to five fractions over one week or 30 Gy in 8–10 fractions over two weeks followed by immediate surgery. For post-operative XRT, 45 Gy in 20 fractions over four to five weeks was recommended, with the course beginning between 30 and 60 days post-operatively. Although a number of XRT schedules were permitted, the most commonly used pre-operative schedule in AXIS was 25 Gy in five fractions: the majority of the remaining patients received 20 Gy in four or five fractions.

One thousand patients, randomised with respect to peri-operative XRT, would be sufficient to detect a 10 per cent improvement due to XRT. It was intended that patients randomised with respect to XRT in AXIS should contribute a reasonably substantial body of data to the world literature on XRT, and particularly its impact on survival, rather than expecting that the AXIS results alone would be definitive. Radiotherapy randomisations peaked in 1991 and declined steadily thereafter through increasing use of elective XRT. The ratio of 1:2 pre- to post-operative XRT was maintained throughout the trial. For 264 patients the intention was to give pre-operative XRT if allocated, and for 497 post-operative XRT was planned. The majority of these patients (87 per cent) were also randomised with respect to 5-FU.

Ninety-nine per cent of pre-operative XRT patients had adenocarcinoma confirmed. Eight patients allocated no pre-operative XRT and 2 of those allocated pre-operative XRT did not have a resection: 9 and 8 per cent respectively were found to have Dukes' A tumours; the proportion of Dukes' B and C tumours was similar across the treatment groups. The proportions considered to have curative resections were 72 and 74 per cent respectively.

As would be expected for the post-operative XRT patients, operative characteristics were well balanced with 99 per cent having adenocarcinoma confirmed, 98 per cent having a resection, and approximately 80 per cent being considered to have had a curative resection.

Implications for future studies

Variations in entry requirements by node status

Most trials of PVI have randomised prior to surgery between PVI and a no-treatment arm. Such trials include node-negative patients since PVI is delivered, of necessity, before the pathology report is available. Published data suggest that the effectiveness of adjuvant treatment in node-negative colorectal cancer is less than for node-positive, and different policies have arisen for the two groups. Some trials (Taylor *et al.* 1985; Wolmark *et al.* 1990) show a benefit for node-negative patients. Modern randomised clinical trials of adjuvant chemotherapy in colorectal cancer distinguish node-positive from node-negative patients. Consensus statements suggest it is now unethical to include a no-treatment arm for node-positive patients. Accrual to the AXIS trial fell off for this reason (Figures 3.2 and 3.3). Future trials of PVI will have to deal with criticisms about over- or under-treatment, depending on the trial methodology.

Sample size

Modern trials of adjuvant systemic chemotherapy separate rectal from colon cancer patients. Rectal, but not colon, cancer patients may require peri-operative pelvic XRT. Modern colon cancer adjuvant studies are usually powered for equivalence between two chemotherapy strategies. Approximately 4,000 patients are required in order to detect an absolute survival improvement at five years of 5 per cent (from 50 to 55 per cent), with 90 per cent power at a two-sided significance level of 5 per cent. Many adjuvant systemic and PVI trials fall below this level of accrual. Because of

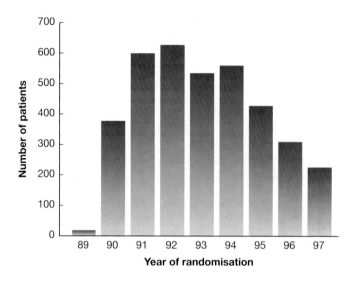

Figure 3.2 Accrual to AXIS by year

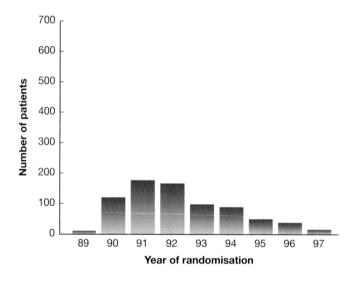

Figure 3.3 Accrual to radiotherapy randomisation in AXIS by year

the interventional nature of PVI, difficulties in compliance and randomisation, large trials are less likely for PVI than for systemic chemotherapy.

Higher doses of 5-FU: new drugs

Protocol drug doses for adjuvant PVI trials were designed to be effective against microscopic rather than established metastases, but dose-intensity may influence outcome. Much higher doses of 5-FU can be used by intra-arterial hepatic infusion and doses can be modulated by concomitant intravenous folinic acid. However, intra-arterial chemotherapy is more costly in terms of time and experience than PVI.

5-FU alone is no longer the most effective treatment for colorectal cancer. Combination schedules of 5-FU with oxaliplatin and irinotecan are now registered as optimal first-line treatment for metastatic disease and adjuvant trials are in progress. Although research continues on strategies for intra-hepatic chemotherapy using drugs other than 5-FU, previous experience suggests that hepatic toxicity might be problematic.

Chemotherapy compliance

Surgical variation

PVI training is not required for specialist accreditation and newly appointed surgeons are unlikely to learn the technique outside a clinical trial. Increasing regulation has made it more difficult for surgeons, who may not be accredited as oncologists, to deliver cytotoxic drugs.

There is some evidence that chemotherapy compliance is more operator-dependent in trials of PVI than in trials of intravenous adjuvant chemotherapy. Technical problems prevent PVI cannulation in around 5 per cent of patients. Although portal cannulation, once learned, adds little to the operation, there is a considerable learning curve. Failure to start the infusion because of technical problems with cannulation and operative complications are less likely with experienced surgeons.

In AXIS, 166 surgeons from seven countries participated; eight surgeons entered more than 100 patients each, and together they contributed 35 per cent of the total number of patients. Fourteen surgeons entered between 51 and 100 patients, and contributed 26 per cent of the total; a further 14 entered between 26 and 50 and contributed 14 per cent of the total, while the 131 surgeons entering 25 or fewer patients contributed 25 per cent of the total. Seventy-four per cent of patients allocated 5-FU began the infusion, and 88 per cent of those who started the infusion completed the full seven days.

Pre- versus intra-operative randomisation, unresected disease: effects on compliance

Many patients with colon cancer do not have a histological diagnosis prior to surgery, and 30 per cent present as an emergency admission. Many trials of PVI have randomised prior to laparotomy, without a histological diagnosis of colorectal carcinoma. Patients were presumed to have colorectal cancer and were excluded from randomisation only if they have a contraindication to receive the protocol treatments. Most published trials were carried out at a time when routine pre-operative detection of liver metastases using CT scanning or staging of rectal cancer using pelvic MRI was unusual.

The PVI trials of adjuvant chemotherapy illustrate a number of methodological problems associated with pre-operative randomisation. Protocol drug doses for adjuvant PVI trials were designed to be effective against microscopic rather than established metastases. For this reason many trials have excluded from analysis the 30 per cent of randomised patients found to have liver metastases or inoperable disease at laparotomy. When such patients are evenly distributed between control or treatment arms and when subsequent palliative chemotherapy is standardised, such an exclusion is unlikely to bias trial analysis. However, it is more likely to detect an advantage to treatment than an intention-to-treat analysis of all randomised patients.

In AXIS approximately 40 per cent of patients were randomised on the day of their operation (though not necessarily intra-operatively, as this information was not recorded). Consequently, 130 patients, 3.7 per cent of the total, were found to have benign disease, while 82 (2.3 per cent) were considered inoperable and did not undergo resection. A further, more substantial group of patients undergoing resection (10.6 per cent of the total) had distant metastases discovered at the time of surgery. All these patients were fairly evenly balanced between the two treatment groups.

Of those randomised to PVI who did not start PVI, the main reasons were inappropriate disease stage – advanced disease or benign disease. However, in the group with confirmed adenocarcinoma who underwent a curative resection, 84 per cent started the infusion and 88 per cent of those that started completed the full seven days.

The effect of pre-operative randomisation on compliance was striking in the XRT randomisation of AXIS. Effectively, AXIS became a comparison of no XRT versus selective post-operative XRT, due to pre-operative randomisation. As with post-operative PVI, a large proportion (36 per cent) of patients randomised to post-operative XRT did not receive it. The primary reason was the discovery of Dukes' A tumours (although the protocol allowed XRT in such cases at the clinician's discretion) or metastatic disease at operation. In contrast, of 132 patients allocated pre-operative XRT, 119 (90 per cent) received treatment according to intent. Nine patients (7 per cent) did not receive any XRT. Pre-treatment (but post-randomisation) investigations led to the discovery of metastatic disease in one and benign disease in another. Three patients, having previously given consent, later refused XRT and a further three died before XRT began.

Pre-operative randomisation can also influence compliance by altering the spectrum of treatment-related morbidity. In published trials of peri-operative XRT for rectal cancer, curatively resected patients allocated post-operative radiotherapy are less compliant than those allocated pre-operative XRT. The main reasons are post-operative complications, including early death and general deterioration. In the AXIS trial, of 248 allocated post-operative XRT, only 134 (54 per cent) received the intended dose (generally 40–45 Gy in 20 fractions), although 32 of these patients started XRT later than planned. Radiation enteritis caused an interruption to one patient's course, and the early termination of two others.

In contrast, there were no reports in AXIS of morbidity sufficient to change the planned pre-operative XRT schedule. The total number of patients with serious complications reported was slightly higher in those allocated XRT (20 versus 11 per cent), bowel obstruction and perineal wound complications being slightly more common, but no complication was statistically significantly raised and there were four post-operative deaths in each group.

Conclusion

The survival results of the AXIS trial, which will be published in the near future, will make a major impact on the acceptability of PVI. AXIS was probably the last multicentre collaborative adjuvant study to randomise both rectal and colon cancer patients as well as Dukes' A, B and C patients. The trial illustrates some of the defects inherent in pre-surgical randomisation and the abscence of pre-surgical CT scanning. However, surgical intervention remains pivotal to the treatment of this disease and it is likely that novel surgical techniques such as PVI will continue to be important.

References

Beart RW, Moertel CG, Wiend HS *et al.* (1990). Adjuvant therapy for resectable colorectal carcinoma with fluorouracil administered by portal vein infusion. *Archives of Surgery* **125**, 897–901.

Fielding LP, Hittinger R, Grace RH *et al.* (1992). Randomised controlled trial of adjuvant chemotherapy by portal-vein infusion after curative resection for colorectal adenocarcinoma. *Lancet* **340**, 502–6.

Goldberg JA, Kerr DJ, Wilmott N *et al.* (1988). Pharmacokinetics and pharmacodynamics of locoregional 5 fluorouracil (5FU) in advanced colorectal liver metastases. *British Journal of Cancer* **57**, 186–9.

Gray R, James R, Mossman J, Stenning S (1991). AXIS – a suitable case for treatment. UKCCCR Colorectal Subcommittee. *British Journal of Cancer* **63**, 841–45.

Holden WD & Dixon WJ (1962). A study on the use of triethylenethiophosphoramide as an adjuvant to surgery in the treatment of colorectal cancer. *Cancer Chemotherapy Reports* **16**, 129–34.

James RD on behalf of the AXIS collaborators (1999). Intraportal 5FU (PVI) and peri-operative radiotherapy (RT) in the adjuvant treatment of colorectal cancer – 3681 patients randomised in the UKCCCR AXIS Trial. *Proceedings of the American Society of Clinical Oncology* **18**, 1013 (abstr.).

Laffer U, Maibach R, Metzger U *et al.* (1998). Randomized trial of adjuvant perioperative chemotherapy in radically resected colorectal cancer (SAKK 40/87). *Proceedings of the American Society of Clinical Oncology* **17**, 983 (abstr.).

Liver Infusion Meta-Analysis Group (1997). Portal vein chemotherapy for colorectal cancer: a meta-analysis of 4,000 patients in 10 studies. *Journal of the National Cancer Institute* **89**, 497–505.

Metzger U, Mermillod B, Aeberhard P *et al.* (1987). Intraportal chemotherapy in colorectal carcinoma as an adjuvant modality. *World Journal of Surgery* **11**, 452–8.

Moertel CG, Fleming TR, Macdonald JS *et al.* (1995). Fluorouracil plus levamisole as effective adjuvant therapy after resection of stage III colon carcinoma. *Annals of Internal medicine* **122**, 321–6.

Morales F, Bell M, McDonald GO *et al.* (1957). The prophylactic treatment of cancer at the time of operation. *Annals of Surgery* **146**, 588–95.

Rougier P, Sahmoud T, Nitti D *et al.* (1998). Adjuvant portal-vein infusion of fluorouracil and heparin in colorectal cancer: a randomised trial. *Lancet* **351**, 1677–81.

[SAKK] Swiss Group for Clinical Cancer Research (1995). Long term results of single course of adjuvant intraportal chemotherapy for colorectal cancer. *Lancet* **345**, 349–53.

Taylor I, Machin D, Mullee M *et al.* (1985). A randomised controlled trial of adjuvant portal vein cytotoxic perfusion in colorectal cancer. *British Journal of Surgery* **72**, 359–63.

Wereldsma JC, Bruggiok ED, Meijer WS *et al.* (1990). Adjuvant portal liver infusion in colorectal cancer with 5-fluorouracil/heparin versus urokinase versus control. Results of a prospective randomised clinical trial. *Cancer* **65**, 425–32.

Wolmark N, Rockette H, Wickerham DL *et al.* (1990). Adjuvant therapy of Dukes' A, B and C adenocarcinoma of the colon with portal vein fluorouracil hepatic infusion: preliminary results of National Surgical Adjuvant Breast and Bowel Project Protocol C-02. *Journal of Clinical Oncology* **8**, 1466–75.

PART 2

Advanced colorectal disease

Chapter 4

Optimal strategies for use of the oral fluoropyrimidines

Donald Bissett, Fareeda Ahmed, Howard McLeod and Jim Cassidy

Introduction

After dominating the cytotoxic treatment of colorectal cancer for almost 40 years, 5-fluorouracil (5-FU) may soon be overtaken by the oral fluoropyrimidines (Figure 4.1), which are being developed for this key role. The schedule-dependency of many biological effects of 5-FU is well established. Bolus 5-FU chemotherapy as a single agent has only modest activity in advanced colorectal cancer, and its dose-limiting toxicities include myelosuppression, nausea and diarrhoea. Continuous-infusion 5-FU provides superior single-agent response rates in colorectal cancer, but with low

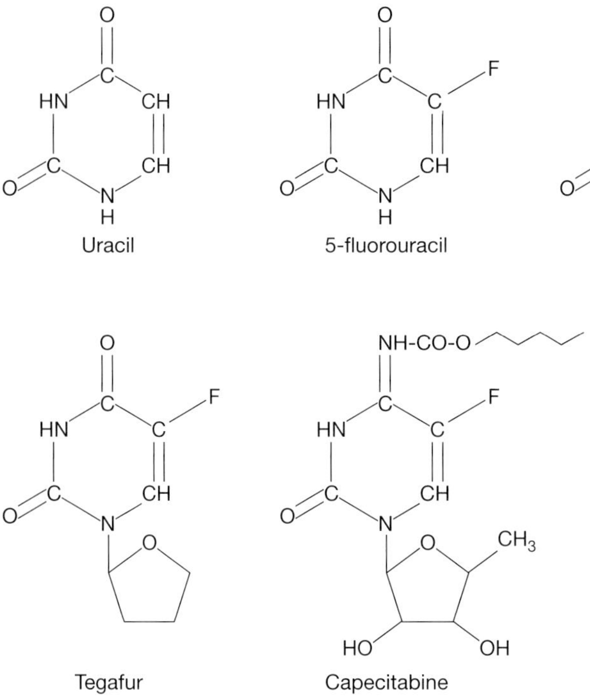

Figure 4.1 Chemical structures of uracil, eniluracil, and the fluoropyrimidines

levels of myelosuppression; however it is associated with significant toxicity, including diarrhoea, mucositis and hand-foot syndrome, and it is also inconvenient because it requires prolonged venous access and an ambulatory pump. The potential of oral fluoropyrimidines as a substitute for prolonged infusion 5-FU was recognised in the 1970s, but it is only now that this promise is being fully realised. This review examines the recent progress made in this field.

Biochemical pathways of 5-FU

The major biological effects of 5-FU are caused by its inhibition of thymidylate synthase, a key enzyme in DNA synthesis (Figure 4.2). The modulation of 5-FU effects by leucovorin (LV) is attributed to the formation of a stabilised complex of thymidylate synthase, 5-fluorodeoxyuridine monophosphate (5dUMP), and reduced folate (Sobrero *et al.* 1997). Incorporation of FUTP or dFUTP into RNA and DNA is also a potential mechanism of cytotoxicity. Protracted infusions of low-dose 5-FU appear to provide antitumour activity comparable with leucovorin-modulated bolus or infusional 5-FU (Leichman *et al.* 1995).

An attractive alternative is the continuous delivery of low-dose fluoropyrimidines by the oral route. Ideally, an oral fluoropyrimidine would have excellent absorption and a half-life of at least several hours to facilitate delivery of a fairly constant

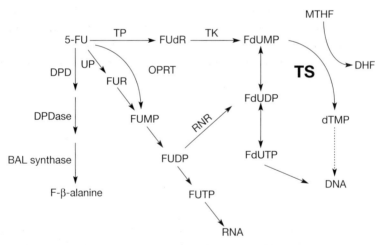

BAL synthase-β-alanine synthase, DHF-dihydrofolate, DPD-dihydropyrimidine dehydrogenase, DPDase-dihdropyrimidinase, MTHF-methyl tetrahydrofolate, OPRT-orotate phosphoribosyltransferase, RNR-ribonucleotide reductase, TK-thymidine kinase, TP-thymidine phosphorylase, TS-thymidylate synthase, UP-uridine phosphorylase

Figure 4.2 Biochemical pathways for 5-FU

systemic concentration of drug. Oral 5-FU itself is a poor candidate for this role. Pharmacokinetic studies of 5-FU have shown that the bioavailability of the drug is unpredictable, ranging from 0 to 80 per cent, with large inter- and intra-patient variations (Fraile *et al*. 1980). The key enzyme in the metabolism of 5-FU is dihydropyrimidine dehydrogenase (DPD), and it is estimated to account for the breakdown of more than 80 per cent of 5-FU (Heggie *et al*. 1987). It is likely that the unpredictability of absorption of 5-FU is due to the variable expression of intestinal and hepatic DPD (McLeod *et al*. 1998). The plasma half-life of 5-FU is short, around ten minutes. Thus oral 5-FU has no useful clinical role in the treatment of colorectal cancer, at least as a single agent.

Eniluracil

Since DPD is the rate-limiting enzyme in the breakdown of 5-FU and accounts for much of the inter-patient variability in metabolism of this agent, it is a logical target for novel therapeutic strategies. Eniluracil is a potent inactivator of DPD. In patients with colorectal cancer, treatment with three days of eniluracil (10 mg bd orally) reduced DPD activity to undetectable levels in normal tissue (white blood cells and colonic mucosa) and in tumour (Figures 4.3 and 4.4) (Ahmed *et al*. 1999). At these doses eniluracil causes elevation of plasma uracil, as expected, but is non-toxic and has no antitumour activity. When 5-FU is administered orally with eniluracil, the pharmacology of 5-FU is dramatically altered. Early clinical trials showed that the maximum tolerable dose (MTD) of 5-FU with eniluracil is only 1.8 mg/m^2 bd, 100 times less than the MTD for continuous-infusion 5-FU (Schilsky *et al*. 1998). The absorption of 5-FU becomes predictable and the half-life of 5-FU is extended from ten minutes to four to five hours (Baker *et al*. 1996). The toxicities of this combination are predictably similar to continuous-infusion 5-FU, namely

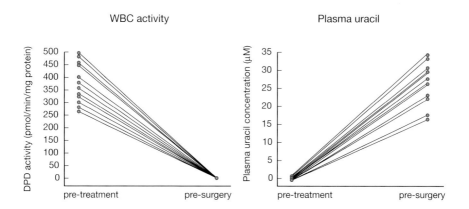

Figure 4.3 Systemic inactivation of DPD in normal tissues by eniluracil

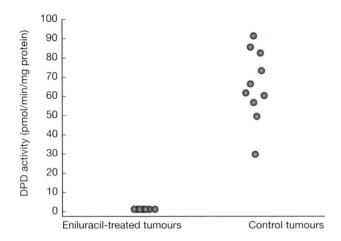

Figure 4.4 Inactivation of DPD in colorectal cancers by eniluracil

diarrhoea, nausea and mucositis. Hand-foot syndrome occurs infrequently and is not severe. Significant neutropenia is rare.

A phase II study of eniluracil and oral 5-FU was conducted in previously untreated metastatic colorectal cancer (Mani *et al.* 1998). Initially, patients were treated with 10 mg bd eniluracil and 1 mg/m^2 bd oral 5-FU for four weeks followed by a single week's break. Low levels of toxicity were observed and a second cohort of patients was treated with a 10 per cent dose increase. The results of the trial are summarised in Table 4.1. The response rate was promising, 27 per cent in 49 assessable patients. The estimated median time to progression was 5.4 months. The treatment was generally well tolerated and myelosuppression was infrequent, with grade 3 neutropenia in only two patients. Diarrhoea was the most frequent toxicity, with grade 3–4 diarrhoea occurring in 20 per cent of the patients treated at the higher dose. It occurred towards the end of the first or second course and generally responded to either treatment with loperamide or a single 20 per cent dose reduction in 5-FU. Two patients had grade 3–4 vomiting, but no patients had grade 3 mucositis and only one patient had hand-foot syndrome. However, two patients did have neurological toxicity – ataxia in one, nystagmus in the other; these are rare toxicities with continuous-infusion 5-FU.

In view of these promising results, a randomised trial has been conducted in untreated metastatic colorectal cancer, comparing eniluracil and oral 5-FU against the Mayo regimen of bolus 5-FU and leucovorin. This study has completed accrual and should report in 2000.

Table 4.1 Phase II study of oral eniluracil and 5-fluorouracil in metastatic colorectal cancer

Dose of 5-FU (mg/m²)	Number of subjects	Number of courses	Number (%) subjects dose reduced	Number (%) courses at starting dose	Number (%) of subjects with G3–4 diarrhoea	Objective response rate (%)
1.0	30	130	6 (20%)	111 (85%)	3 (10%)	25
1.15	25	89	7 (26%)	80 (90%)	5 (20%)	29
Total	55	219	13 (24%)	191 (87%)	8 (14.5%)	27

Source: Mani *et al.* (1998)

Uracil-ftorafur

Ftorafur is a pro-drug of 5-FU, developed in the 1960s. It is slowly converted to 5-FU by cytochrome P450, thus avoiding breakdown by DPD in the small bowel. As a single agent it has modest activity in colorectal cancer. When combined with uracil in a 1:4 ratio (UFT), the uracil competes for DPD, thereby further increasing the systemic delivery of 5-FU. The plasma half-life of 5-FU is extended to seven hours. This combination was developed in 1978 in Japan and has subsequently been investigated in the US and Europe using a variety of schedules (Sulkes *et al.* 1998). Phase II studies of UFT in colorectal cancer have shown response rates of 17–26 per cent. Subsequent attempts to improve on this have concentrated on the modulation of UFT activity by leucovorin. Pazdur *et al.* (1994) reported a response rate of 42 per cent in a phase II study of 56 untreated patients with metastatic colorectal cancer, receiving UFT 300–350 mg/m²/day and LV 150 mg/day d1-28 q5/52. The higher dose level of UFT caused unacceptable toxicity. The major toxicities of UFT with or without LV are diarrhoea, nausea and mucositis. However, some trials have also reported dose-limiting myelosuppression, and there have been sporadic cases of cutaneous and neurological toxicity.

Two large phase III studies of UFT-LV versus 5-FU-LV were reported at ASCO 1999. The study designs and results are summarised in Table 4.2. The UFT-LV regimen in both was UFT 300 mg/m²/d and LV 75 or 90 mg/d, d1-28, q5/52. Pazdur *et al.* (1999) compared the UFT-LV with the Mayo regimen (bolus 5-FU 425mg/m² and leucovorin 20mg/m², d1-5, q4/52) in 816 patients with untreated metastatic colorectal cancer. Although the response rate was lower in the 5-FU arm (11 versus 15 per cent) this did not reach statistical significance, and the time to progression and overall survival were similar for the two arms. The UFT-LV regimen was better tolerated with significantly less mucositis and myelosuppression, and similar rates of grade 3–4 diarrhoea. Interestingly, no significant hand-foot syndrome was recorded.

Table 4.2 Phase III studies of UFT-LV versus 5-FU-LV in metastatic colorectal cancer

	Pazdur et al. 816 patients		Carmichael et al. 380 patients	
	UFT-LV	5-FU/LV	UFT-LV	5-FU/LV
Response rate (%)	11	15	11	9
Median time to progression (mths)	3.5	3.8	3.4	3.3
Median survival time (mths)	12.4	13.4	12.3	10.3
G3–4 toxicities (%):				
Diarrhoea	21	16	18	11
Mucositis	1	20	2	16
Neutropenia	1	56	3	31

Sources: Carmichael *et al.* (1999); Pazdur *et al.* (1999)

The Carmichael *et al.* (1999) study used as its comparator arm a less intensive regimen, with the same dose of 5-FU and LV given at 5-week intervals. Perhaps not surprisingly, the response rates in both arms of this study were low (UFT-LV 11 per cent, 5-FU-LV 9 per cent), and the survival times similar. Again the UFT-LV regimen was associated with less mucositis and myelosuppression, although diarrhoea was more frequent with UFT-LV, and hand-foot syndrome was uncommon and mild. Both studies conclude that UFT-LV is a more convenient and safe alternative to bolus 5-FU-LV in this setting.

A number of studies of adjuvant therapy with unmodulated UFT in resected colorectal cancer have shown benefit compared with no chemotherapy (Sulkes *et al.* 1998). Large phase III randomised studies of UFT-LV versus 5-FU-LV in the adjuvant setting are ongoing, or recently completed.

Capecitabine

Capecitabine was designed as an oral tumour-selective fluoropyrimidine. The inactive pro-drug is well- and reliably absorbed unchanged and is metabolised in the liver to 5'-deoxy-5-fluorocytidine (DFCR). This is converted to 5'-deoxy-5-fluorouridine (DFUR) by cytidine deaminase, in the liver and in tumour. The third step is the conversion of DFUR to 5-FU by thymidine phosphorylase, and it is this enzyme which is preferentially overexpressed in tumour, leading to tumour-selective exposure to 5-FU. Clinical studies have confirmed this therapeutic targeting (Schuller *et al.* 1997). A group of patients with colorectal cancer undergoing elective resection of either the primary lesion or liver metastases were treated with capecitabine (1,225 mg/m^2/d) for five to seven days prior to surgery. Fluoropyrimidine levels were measured in the resected tumour, adjacent normal tissue, and plasma. The results, expressed as the ratio of tumour to normal tissue 5-FU concentration, confirmed the preferential delivery of 5-FU to the tumour with higher selectivity in primary colorectal tumours compared with liver metastases (Table 4.3).

Table 4.3 Tumour selectivity of capecitabine in resected colorectal cancers and metastases

	Colorectal resections			Hepatic resections		
	Tumour/ normal tissue	Tumour/ plasma	Normal tissue/ plasma	Metastasis/ normal liver	Metastasis/ plasma	Normal liver/ plasma
Mean	3.21*	21.4	8.85	1.41	9.94	7.89
Maximum	8.02	59.9	25.9	2.67	23.6	14.1
N	11	8	8	11	8	8

* Selectivity is expressed as the ratio of the 5-FU concentration between two tissues

Source: Schuller *et al.* (1997)

The phase I and II studies of capecitabine evaluated both continuous and intermittent (d1-14, q3/52) schedules, with and without LV modulation. The results of the randomised phase II study in colorectal cancer are summarised in Table 4.4. All three schedules showed promising antitumour activity. The major toxicities of capecitabine were diarrhoea, hand-foot syndrome, nausea and mucositis. The addition of LV increased toxicity, in particular diarrhoea and hand-foot syndrome, without any perceptible increase in antitumour efficacy. During these early clinical trials of capecitabine it became clear that grade 3–4 toxicities could often be avoided by interrupting therapy when grade 2 diarrhoea or hand-foot syndrome first occurred, and re-introducing capecitabine when non-haematological toxicities had resolved to grade 0-1. A specific grading system for hand-foot syndrome was derived during the clinical development of this compound (Table 4.5).

Table 4.4 Phase II trial of three capecitabine schedules in metastatic colorectal cancer

Schedule of capecitabine	Dose of capecitabine (mg/m²/d)	N	Response rate (%)	Grade 3–4 toxicities (%)		
				Diarrhoea	Hand-foot	Mucositis
Continuous no LV	1,331	37	22	5	10	0
Intermittent no LV	2,510	32	25	9	15	3
Intermittent + LV*	1,657	33	24	20	23	3

* Dose of leucovorin was 30 mg bd

Source: Findlay *et al.* (1997)

Table 4.5 Grading of hand-and-foot syndrome in capecitabine studies

Grade	Clinical domain	Functional domain
1*	Numbness, dysaesthesia, tingling, painless swelling, or erythema	Discomfort which does not disrupt normal activities
2	Painful erythema with swelling	Discomfort which affects activities of daily living
3	Moist desquamation, ulceration, blistering, severe pain	Severe discomfort, unable to work or perform activities of daily living

* Grade is assigned from the domain for which patient scores worst

Two large randomised phase III studies of intermittent capecitabine (2,500 mg/m^2/d d1-14, q3/52) versus the Mayo regimen of bolus 5-FU-LV (5-FU 450 mg/m^2 and LV 20 mg/m^2 d1-5, q4/52) were conducted in advanced colorectal cancer, and these also reported at ASCO 1999. In the study by Twelves *et al.* (1999), 602 patients were randomised (Table 4.6). The response rates, time to progression and overall survival were not significantly different in the two arms. The frequency of grade 3–4 diarrhoea was similar in both arms, but the 5-FU-LV regimen was associated with considerably more grade 3–4 mucositis and neutropenia, and dose reductions were required in 35 per cent of patients. Grade 3 hand-foot syndrome did occur in 16.2 per cent of the capecitabine arm, compared with less than 1 per cent of the 5-FU-LV patients. Dose reductions were required in 27 per cent of capecitabine patients.

In the study of Cox *et al.* with 605 patients there was an advantage in terms of improved response rate in the capecitabine arm (27.1 versus 17.3 per cent), although the time to progression and overall survival in the two arms were similar (Table 4.6). Again, the safety profile favoured capecitabine with similar rates of grade 3–4 diarrhoea, but increased neutropenia and stomatitis in the 5-FU-LV arm. Grade 3 hand-foot syndrome occurred in 17.7 per cent of the capecitabine patients; 40 per cent of the capecitabine and 45 per cent 5-FU-LV patients required dose reductions.

From these studies it is clear that capecitabine is a safe, tolerable and convenient alternative to conventional bolus 5-FU-LV. Its role in the adjuvant therapy of resectable colon cancer is currently being examined in randomised trials against 5-FU-LV.

Conclusion

A number of strategies are now available utilising oral fluoropyrimidines, which offer a safe and tolerable alternative to conventional bolus 5-FU-LV regimens in the treatment of metastatic colorectal cancer. Although no large randomised studies have compared these treatments with either continuous low-dose infusional 5-FU or leucovorin-modulated infusional 5-FU (such as the de Gramont regimen), it seems unlikely that a major difference in efficacy exists. At present, there are only hints to

Table 4.6 Phase III studies of capecitabine versus 5-FU-LV in metastatic colorectal cancer

	Twelves et al. 602 patients		*Cox* et al. 605 patients	
	Capecitabine	*5-FU/LV*	*Capecitabine*	*5-FU/LV*
Response rate (%)	21.1	16.1	27.1	17.3
Median time to progression (mths)	5.5	4.9	4.4	5.1
Median survival time (mths)	13.7	13.0	–	–
G3–4 toxicities (%):				
Diarrhoea	10.7	10.4	15.1	13.9
Mucositis	1	20	–	16.3
Neutropenia	2	19.7	–	25.9
Hand-foot	16.2	0.3	17.7	0

Sources: Cox *et al.* (1999); Twelves *et al.* (1999

guide which might be the best strategy with oral fluoropyrimidines, and indeed there may be good reason to select different strategies for individual patients.

The problem of hand-foot syndrome is intriguing. It does appear that blockade of DPD, either by eniluracil or uracil itself, is associated with reduced cutaneous toxicity, despite exposure of other normal tissues and tumour to levels of 5-FU sufficient to cause significant and predicted effects. It has been suggested that the major cause of hand-foot syndrome may not be 5-FU but rather the metabolic product of DPD, fluoro-β-alanine (Spector *et al.* 1995). This remains to be confirmed.

Although hand-foot syndrome is common with capecitabine, in the majority of cases it is easily managed. Capecitabine does, at present, have a most encouraging record of antitumour activity in colorectal cancer. It is likely that the tumour-selectivity of this drug is relevant to this, and capecitabine uniquely offers potential for selection of patients most likely to gain from this because of overexpression of thymidine phosphorylase in their tumour.

What is clear is that the oral fluoropyrimidines offer superior tolerability compared with conventional bolus 5-FU regimens. Although the adjuvant studies of UFT-LV and capecitabine are still ongoing, it seems inevitable that the use of these agents in both advanced and resected colorectal cancer will rapidly increase over the next few years. Nonetheless, there is an imperative that clinical trials continue to address fundamental uncertainties in the management of this disease, not least the optimum duration of adjuvant therapy and the role of adjuvant fluoropyrimidines in resected rectal cancer.

More exciting is the prospect of combining oral fluoropyrimidines with new agents active in colorectal cancer, such as irinotecan and oxaliplatin. Early clinical experience had already shown these combinations to be feasible, although they do present difficulties in the design of schedules because of the variety of options in terms of both the timing and duration of the fluoropyrimidine component. A further rich vein for clinical investigation is likely to be the use of oral fluoropyrimidines in chemoirradiation, and studies in rectal cancer are already ongoing.

References

Ahmed FY, Johnston SJ, Cassidy J, O'Kelly T, Binnie N, Murray GI, van Gennip AH, Abeling NGGM, Knight S & McLeod HL (1999). Eniluracil treatment completely inactivates dihydropyrimidine dehydrogenase activity in colorectal tumours. *Journal of Clinical Oncology* **17**, 1–7.

Baker SD, Khor SP, Adjei AA, Doucette M, Spector T, Donehower RC, Grochow LB, Sartorius SE, Noe DA, Hohneker JA & Rowinsky EK (1996). Pharmacokinetic, oral bioavailability, and safety study of fluorouracil in patients treated with 776C85, an inactivator of dihydropyrimidine dehydrogenase. *Journal of Clinical Oncology* **14**, 3085–96.

Carmichael J, Popiela T, Radstone D, Falk S, Fey M, Oza A, Skovsgaard T & Martin C (1999). Randomised comparative study of ORZEL® (oral uracil/tegafur) plus leucovorin versus parenteral 5-fluorouracil plus leucovorin in patients with metastatic colorectal cancer. *Proceedings of the American Society of Clinical Oncology* **18**, 1015.

Cox JV, Pazdur R, Thibault A, Maroun J, Weaver C, Jahn MW, Harrison E & Griffin T (1999). A phase III trial of Xeloda™ (capecitabine) in previously untreated advanced / metastatic colorectal cancer. *Proceedings of the American Society of Clinical Oncology* **18**, 1016.

Findlay M, van Cutsem E, Kocha W, Allman D, Laffranchi B, Griffin T, Osterwalder B, Dalley D, Pazdur R & Verweij J (1997). A randomised phase II study of Xeloda™ (capecitabine) in patients with advanced colorectal cancer. *Proceedings of the American Society of Clinical Oncology* **16**, 798.

Fraile RJ, Baker LH, Buroker TR, Horwitz J & Vaitkevicius VK (1980). Pharmacokinetics of 5-fluorouracil administered orally, by rapid intravenous and by slow infusion. *Cancer Research* **40**, 2223–8.

Heggie GD, Sommadossi JP, Cross DS, Huster WJ & Diasio RB (1987). Clinical pharmacokinetics of 5-fluorouracil and its metabolites in plasma, urine, and bile. *Cancer Research* **47**, 2203–6.

Leichman CG, Fleming TR, Muggia FM, Tangen CM, Ardalan B, Doroshow JH, Meyers FJ, Holcombe RF, Weiss GR, Mangalik A *et al.* (1995). Phase II study of fluorouracil and its modulation in advanced colorectal cancer: a Southwest Oncology Group study. *Journal of Clinical Oncology* **13**, 1303–11.

Mani S, Beck T, Chevlen E, Hochster H, O'Rourke M, Weaver C, Bell W, McGuirt C, Levin J, Hohneker J & Lokich J (1998). A phase II open-label study to evaluate a 28-day regimen of oral 5-fluorouracil plus 776C85 (eniluracil) for the treatment of patients with previously untreated metastatic colorectal cancer. *Proceedings of the American Society of Clinical Oncology* **17**, 1083.

McLeod HJ, Sludden J, Murray GI, Keenan RA, Davidson AL, Park K, Koruth M & Cassidy J (1998). Characterisation of dihydropyrimidine dehydrogenase in human colorectal tumours. *British Journal of Cancer* **77**, 461–5.

Pazdur R, Lassere Y, Rhodes V, Ajani JA, Sugarman SM, Patt YZ, Jones DV Jr, Markowitz AB, Abbruzzese JL & Bready B (1994). Phase II trial of uracil and tegafur plus oral leucovorin: an effective oral regimen in the treatment of metastatic colorectal carcinoma. *Journal of Clinical Oncology* **12**, 2296–300.

Pazdur R, Douillard J-Y, Skillings JR, Eisenberg PD, Davidson N, Harper P, Vincent MD, Lembersky BC & Benner SE (1999). Multicentre phase III study of 5-fluorouracil or UFT™ in combination with leucovorin in patients with metastatic colorectal cancer. *Proceedings of the American Society of Clinical Oncology* **18**, 1009.

Schilsky RL, Hohneker J, Ratain MJ, Janisch L, Smetzer L, Lucas VS, Khor SP, Diasio R, von Hoff DD & Burris HA (1998). Phase I clinical and pharmacologic study of eurluracil plus fluorouracil in patients with advanced cancer. *Journal of Clinical Oncology* **16**, 1450–7.

Schuller J, Cassidy J, Reigner BG, Durston R, Roos B, Ishitsuka H, Utoh M & Dumont E (1997). Tumour selectivity of Xeloda™ in colorectal cancer patients. *Proceedings of the American Society of Clinical Oncology* **17**, 797.

Sobrero AF, Aschele C & Bertino JR (1997). Fluorouracil in colorectal cancer – a tale of two drugs: implications for biochemical modulation. *Journal of Clinical Oncology* **15**, 368–81.

Spector T, Cao SS, Rustum YM, Harrington JA & Porter DJT (1995). Attenuation of the antitumour activity of 5-fluorouracil by (R)-5-fluoro-5,6-dihydrouracil. *Cancer Research* **55**, 1239–41.

Sulkes A, Benner SE & Canetta RM (1998). Uracil-ftorafur: an oral fluoropyrimidine active in colorectal cancer. *Journal of Clinical Oncology* **16**, 3461–75.

Twelves C, Harper P, van Cutsem E, Thibault A, Shelygin YA, Burger HU, Allman D & Osterwalder B (1999). A phase III trial of Xeloda™ (capecitabine) in previously untreated advanced/metastatic colorectal cancer. *Proceedings of the American Society of Clinical Oncology* **18**, 1010.

This chapter appears by kind permission of *Clinical Oncology.*

Chapter 5

Combination chemotherapy for advanced colorectal cancer

Matthew T Seymour

Introduction

For most of the last three decades, the development of chemotherapy for colorectal cancer has been a process of meticulous optimisation of single-agent therapy with 5-fluorouracil (5-FU). Within this straightjacket, considerable progress has been made. Indeed, 5-FU has turned out to be a more active and versatile drug than first imagined: it has a well-established evidence base for benefit in both the adjuvant and palliative setting and, when used well, it lacks many of the distressing side-effects of other cytotoxic drugs.

However, 5-FU also has many limitations. For around a third of patients, not even temporary stabilisation of disease is obtained, and over the past ten years it has become clear that even the most active 5-FU regimens, when subjected to the rigours of well-conducted, externally reviewed, multicentre phase III trials, produce WHO objective partial or complete responses in fewer than 30 per cent of patients.

In the early 1980s Goldie & Coldman (1984) and others developed models of tumour growth and response to chemotherapy incorporating the concepts of genetic and phenotypic instability, with the emergence of drug-resistant clones during treatment. They predicted that the results of chemotherapy would be improved by the use of concurrent or alternating drug schedules, provided the individual agents were (a) independently active, and (b) non-cross-resistant. These ideas have underpinned the development of combination chemotherapy for most cancers, but could not be applied or tested in colorectal cancer since only one active agent, 5-FU, was available.

At last, this situation is changing. Recent years have seen the arrival of two new drugs, oxaliplatin and irinotecan, each with the properties of independent activity and non-cross-resistance, which are pre-requisites for combination therapy in the Goldie-Coldman model. In addition, new evidence has emerged for an old drug, mitomycin, suggesting that it, too, may have a role in combination chemotherapy for colorectal cancer.

In this chapter, we shall review the current evidence for the non-cross resistant activity of these three agents by looking at their use in patients with 5-FU-resistant disease, then examine their role in first-line combination chemotherapy.

Drugs showing non-cross-resistance with 5-FU

Irinotecan (CPT-11; Campto) is a semi-synthetic derivative of camptothecin. Its active metabolite, SN38, causes cytotoxicity through interaction with the endonuclease topoisomerase-I (topo-I). The normal function of topo-I is to relieve torsion which inevitably develops 'upstream' of the replication fork when DNA strands are separating during mitosis or transcription. When DNA is under torsional strain, topo-I binds to it, makes a single strand break and allows the nicked strand to rotate around the intact strand before re-ligating it (see Figure 5.1). SN38 binds to the topo-I-DNA 'cleavable complex', stabilising it and preventing re-ligation. This leads on to double strand breaks when the replication fork collides with the cleavable complex.

The pharmacology of irinotecan, illustrated in Figure 5.2, is important, as several elements may lead to interpatient variability. Clearance of the active metabolite SN38 occurs through glucuronidation by UGT1A1, and biliary excretion of both SN38 and SN38-glucuronide – a process which involves transport systems such as P-glycoprotein and cMOAT. Glucuronidation is reduced in patients with Gilbert's syndrome or Crigler Najjar syndrome, and may be induced by drugs such as phenobarbitone. Biliary excretion may be inhibited by various drugs, including cyclosporin-A, or by physical causes. SN38 in the small bowel may be responsible for the delayed

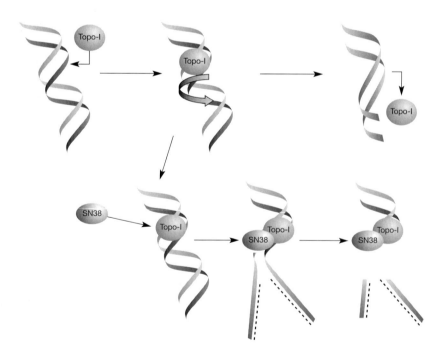

Figure 5.1 Mechanism of action of topoisomerase-I and effect of the irinotecan metabolite SN38 (see text for explanation)

diarrhoea which is one of the dose-limiting toxicities of irinotecan (Ratain 1998; Ratain *et al.* 1999).

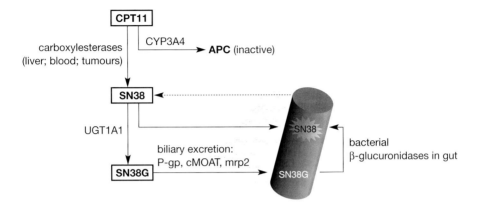

Figure 5.2 Pathways of activation and clearance of irinotecan (see text for explanation)

There is good clinical evidence that irinotecan, as a single agent, is an active drug in patients with 5-FU-resistant disease. Randomised phase III trials of around 270 patients each were reported in 1998, both examining irinotecan at 300–350 mg/m^2 three-weekly for advanced disease progressing during or soon after 5-FU therapy. In one trial the control arm was supportive care alone (Cunningham *et al.* 1998); in the other, an infusional 5-FU regimen (Rougier *et al.* 1998). Both trials showed statistically significant survival advantages in favour of irinotecan with median improvements of 2.7 months (p=0.0001) and 2.3 months (p=0.035), respectively. There is promising evidence that the significant toxicity of the three-weekly schedule used in these phase III trials may be reduced by more frequent dose fractionation, or by pharmacokinetic modulation (Rothenberg *et al.* 1998; Tzavaris *et al.* 1999; Ratain *et al.* 1999). Irinotecan's non-cross-resistance with 5-FU is underlined by the fact that this second-line activity is obtained despite irinotecan being no more active than 5-FU in unpretreated patients (Rougier *et al.* 1997; Saltz *et al.* 1999).

Oxaliplatin (L-OHP; Eloxatin) is a novel organoplatin which forms DNA adducts in a similar manner to cisplatin, but possesses a non-leaving group of diaminocyclohexane (DACH). The adducts formed are therefore distinct from other platins and the activity of the drug, both in pre-clinical models and clinically, is also distinct. One property of DACH-Pt adducts appears to be that, unlike cisplatin adducts, they are neither recognised by, nor dependent for cytotoxicity upon, the mismatch repair (MMR) protein complex (Figure 5.3) (Fink *et al.* 1996). This is of relevance since abnormalities of MMR are common in colorectal cancer and may confer resistance to other drugs such as 5-FU (Barratt *et al.* 1998).

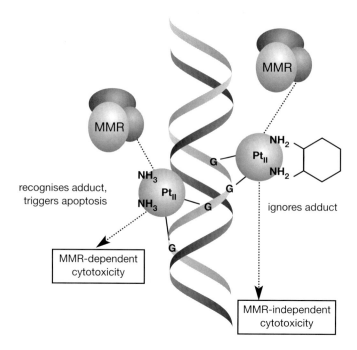

Figure 5.3 Contrasting effect of cisplatin-DNA adduct *(left)* and oxaliplatin-DNA adduct *(right)*. Unlike cisplatin, oxaliplatin adducts are not recognised by, or dependent upon, the mismatch repair (MMR) system

For reasons that are not fully understood, oxaliplatin and 5-FU interact synergistically *in vitro*. Therefore, clinical development of the drug has, from an early stage, concentrated on combinations with 5-FU rather than single-agent therapy. Evidence for non-cross-resistance of these combinations with single-agent 5-FU/FA comes from studies in which patients with documented disease progression on 5-FU/FA alone were treated with oxaliplatin or oxaliplatin/5-FU/FA.

Unlike irinotecan, there has been no phase III randomised trial to quantify the effect of second-line oxaliplatin on survival in this setting; however, phase II data would suggest that its activity is at least as great as irinotecan. Large phase II second-line series include the following:

- single-agent oxaliplatin in 106 patients, with a reported objective response rate (RR) of 10 per cent (Machover *et al.* 1996);
- oxaliplatin added to fortnightly 5-FU bolus plus infusion ('FOLFOX') in around 130 patients, with reported RRs of 20–40 per cent and median survival of 10–16 months from starting second-line therapy (de Gramont *et al.* 1997b; Wilson *et al.* 1998; de Gramont *et al.* 1999);

- oxaliplatin added to chronomodulated 5-FU/FA in 67 patients, with RRs of 29–55 per cent and median survival of 12–17 months (Levi *et al.* 1992; Garufi *et al.* 1995);
- oxaliplatin added to the Mayo Clinic or AIO schedules in 172 patients, with a RR of 11 per cent and median survival of 10.5 months (van Cutsem *et al.* 1999).

These data, although not randomised, are comparable with pooled phase II data for single-agent irinotecan in similar patient populations, where the RR was 13 per cent of 363 patients (c.i. 10–17 per cent) and median survival was 9.5 months (van Cutsem *et al.* 1997).

Mitomycin C has long been used in other gastrointestinal tract cancers, but its role in colorectal cancer is not clear. Three recent small studies have re-evaluated it in 5-FU-resistant disease. Seitz *et al.* (1998) reported a high response rate and median survival of 10 months in 24 5-FU-resistant patients treated with mitomycin plus the bimonthly bolus + infusion 5-FU/FA, and our group obtained similarly good results with protracted venous infusion 5-FU + bolus mitomycin in 26 patients (Chester *et al.* 2000). However, a study of single-agent mitomycin, given by 120-hour infusion, was less encouraging (Hartmann *et al.* 1998).

First-line combination therapy

After demonstrating independent activity against colorectal cancer and non-cross resistance with 5-FU, the next logical step is to develop a combination chemotherapy schedule and compare it with single-agent 5-FU as first-line therapy. A general scheme for these investigations is shown in Figure 5.4. To date, two such trials are reported for irinotecan, two for oxaliplatin and one for mitomycin. The results of all five are summarised in Table 5.1.

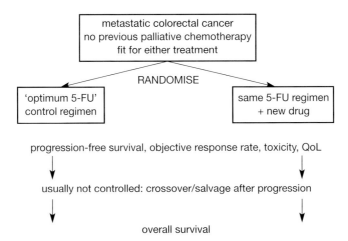

Figure 5.4 General schema for trials of first-line combination chemotherapy

Table 5.1

Reference	Treatment	N	RR (PR+CR)	Median PFS	Median OS
Saltz et al. (1999)	Mayo 5d 5-FU/FA versus weekly 5-FU/FA/	219	22% (p=0.001)	19wk (p=0.008)	12.6 mths (not signif.)
	irinotecan versus	225	40%	30 wks	14.4 mths
	weekly irinotecan	223	18%	18 wks	12.0 mths
Douillard et al. (2000)	5-FU/FA (LV5-FU2 or AIO) versus same 5-FU/FA	187	23% (p<0.001)	19 wks (p<0.001)	14.0 mths (P=0.028)
	+ irinotecan	198	41%	29wks	16.9mths
de Gramont et al. (1998)	5-FU/FA (LV5-FU2) versus same 5-FU/FA	210	22% (p<0.0001)	26wks (p<0.0001)	14.7mths (not signif.)
	+ oxaliplatin	210	50%	38 wks	16.2 mths
Giacchetti et al. (1997)	5-FU/FA (chrono) versus same 5-FU/FA	100	12% (p<0.0001)	23 wks (p<0.05)	19.4 mths (not signif.)
	+ oxaliplatin	100	34%	39 wk	17.6 mths
Ross et al. (1997)	Protracted infusion 5-FU versus same 5-FU	100	38% (p=0.024)	23 wks (p=0.033)	(p=0.033)*
	+ mitomycim	100	54%	34 wks	

* Not significant in the original paper. Updated analysis: Price (1999).

Irinotecan/5-FU combinations

The two trials involving irinotecan were presented at the 1999 ASCO meeting. Both were international, multicentre and large, one from the USA, Canada, Australia and New Zealand (Saltz et al. 1999), the other from Europe (Douillard et al. 2000).

In the American/Antipodean trial (Saltz et al. 1999), 683 patients were randomised to bolus 5-FU/FA alone, irinotecan alone, or an irinotecan + bolus 5-FU/FA combination. The design did not quite conform to the scheme in Figure 5.4, since the 5-FU/FA schedule in the control arm (the Mayo clinic 5-day monthly schedule) differed from the weekly-times 4 schedule used in the combination arm. Neither of these 5-FU schedules can be regarded as 'optimum', the Mayo clinic 'control' regimen having proven substantially inferior to biweekly bolus and infusional 5-FU/FA in a previous phase III trial (de Gramont et al. 1997).

Editorial Note. Subsequent to the original date of publication of this clinical text, Saltz et al. (1999) – see Table 5.1 above – have published their full paper where analyses demonstrate that median OS of weekly 5-FU/FA/irinotecan vs. Mayo 5d 5-FU/FA is 14.8 mths vs 12.6 mths. This represents a statistically significant difference (p=0.04). [Saltz BL et al. (2000). Irinotecan plus fluorouracil and leucovorin for metastatic colorectal cancer. New England Journal of Medicine **343**, 905–14].

Irinotecan causes diarrhoea, neutropenia, myelosuppression and lethargy: one concern, therefore, was whether these overlapping toxicities would make the 5-FU/irinotecan combination too toxic, but this was not the case. In fact, the toxicity of irinotecan plus 5-FU was perhaps even antagonistic: the incidence of grade 3–4 diarrhoea was actually lower in the combination arm (23 per cent of patients) than in the single-agent irinotecan arm (31 per cent), despite using the same dose and schedule of irinotecan. Neutropenia was increased, but was still less than with the Mayo clinic 'control' regimen.

On the other hand, the antitumour effects were clearly not antagonistic: single-agent 5-FU/FA and single-agent irinotecan gave almost identical progression-free survival (PFS) and RR, but results for the combination were significantly improved (see Table 5.1). This benefit did not translate into improved survival, probably because a proportion of patients in the single-agent arms gained benefit from salvage crossover therapy. This trial has subsequently been re-analysed and updated twice, once in an abstract (Saltz *et al.* 2000), then orally. The *p* value for survival has now fallen to 0.046, although the significance of this finding is reduced by the multiple analyses.

The European trial (Douillard *et al.* 2000) involved 387 patients. These investigators wished to use an optimum 5-FU/FA control regimen, but instead of agreeing a single schedule, gave clinicians a choice of using either the French fortnightly bolus + infusion (LV5-FU2) or the German weekly 24-hour infusion (AIO) regimen. With the latter, the dose of 5-FU was reduced in the combination schedule.

The addition of irinotecan significantly increased toxicity compared with 5-FU/FA alone, with neutropenia, fevers, diarrhoea, nausea and asthenia. However, the efficacy was also significantly increased, with improved time to progression and response rate. In this trial, overall survival was also significantly increased despite the fact that 31 per cent of control arm patients received irinotecan-containing salvage therapy, and patients in both arms received alternative drugs.

The two trials of 5-FU/FA ± irinotecan have now been co-analysed. This, predictably, strengthens the statistical significance of the main study endpoints, including survival (Saltz *et al.* 2000).

Oxaliplatin/5-FU combinations

Two trials of the design shown in Figure 5.4 have been reported to date. The larger was first reported at ASCO in 1998 (de Gramont *et al.* 2000) and updated at the 1999 meeting (Seymour *et al.* 1999): 420 patients were randomised to the 'LV5-FU2' fortnightly regimen of bolus and infusional 5-FU/FA with or without the addition of oxaliplatin. The addition of oxaliplatin increased toxicity, although this remained relatively mild. The characteristic toxicity of oxaliplatin is peripheral sensory neuropathy which, although very common, is mild and reversible in the large majority of cases. However, 16 per cent of patients developed grade 3 neuropathy (involving pain or functional loss) and in one quarter of these (4 per cent patients) it was irreversible.

The efficacy of the combination was markedly improved, with highly significant increases in RR and PFS (see Table 5.1). Overall survival was not significantly affected, again perhaps explained by crossover and second-line treatment.

A previous, smaller study of similar design examined the addition of oxaliplatin to chronomodulated 5-FU/FA (Giacchetti 1997). Again, marked increases were seen in RR and PFS, although in this trial the control regimen produced a lower RR than in previous chronotherapy studies. Strangely, the control arm patients in this study enjoyed the longest median overall survival of all the trials reviewed, although the difference between the the two arms was not statistically significant. A high proportion of patients in both arms of this trial had subsequent hepatic surgery, and it is worth noting that 57 per cent of the control patients went on to receive oxaliplatin as second-line therapy. This raises the question of the optimum sequencing of therapies for this disease.

Mitomycin/5-FU combination

Only one trial has asked the same question of mitomycin. It involved 200 patients randomised to continuous ambulatory 5-FU infusion alone or with six-weekly bolus mitomycin. The dose of mitomycin was reduced during the trial to remove the risk of a rare but serious toxicity of this drug, haemolytic uraemic syndrome. This was a single-centre trial, and the response rate of 34 per cent to the control treatment was higher than expected. The combination arm had significantly better RR and failure-free survival. When first reported, survival was not affected (Ross *et al.* 1997), but a recent update now shows a small but significant survival advantage at two years (Price 1999). In a subsequent randomised trial from the same group, 160 control arm patients received the same 5-FU/mitomycin regimen with, once again, encouraging results in terms of failure-free survival (median 36 weeks) and overall survival (median 17.6 months) although RR was lower at 40 per cent (Price 1999).

Conclusions

Until recently, we had only one useful drug for colorectal cancer: 5-FU. Now, 5-FU itself is being challenged by a range of pro-drugs and alternatives, which may soon replace it (see Chapter 4), but more importantly we have at least two new agents with completely different mechanisms of action, which lack cross-resistance and which may feasibly be combined with 5-FU. At long last we have entered the era of combination chemotherapy for colorectal cancer. The obvious next question is how to make best use of this new potential, both for patients with advanced disease and for those being treated with curative intent.

Where cure is a realistic goal, and the aim of chemotherapy is complete clonal eradication of cancer, the lesson from Goldie & Coldman, and from our experience in other cancers, is to use combination chemotherapy. Two-drug combinations as described in this chapter, but perhaps also three or even four-drug combinations, offer exciting potential to cure more patients with conventionally operable disease, and to bring more patients within the scope of curative surgery (see Chapter 2). These schedules must be safe and deliverable without too much compromise to individual-agent dose-intensity, and the ongoing programmes of combination development in patients with advanced disease are the appropriate testing ground to establish new regimens and compare their efficacy. Three of the schedules established in the work reviewed here are already now under test in phase III adjuvant therapy trials.

When cure is not a goal, the aim of chemotherapy is to suppress the cancer burden below the threshold of symptoms and to keep it suppressed for as long as possible – i.e. to achieve the maximum possible extension of survival with good quality of life. It is possible that first-line combination chemotherapy will also be the best strategy to achieve this: the same principle of early suppression of all potentially sensitive clones may also be applied to non-curative therapy. However, this strategy carries a cost, in terms of both finance and toxicity, and will require testing.

If a patient has advanced disease and cure is not a goal, and if we plan to use more than one drug, should we give them together from the start, or use them sequentially? None of the trials reviewed sets out to answer that question, however, those testing first-line oxaliplatin or irinotecan combinations had 27–57 per cent of control arm patients who crossed over to receive the test drug on progression. In one trial (Douillard *et al.* 2000), and possibly a second (Saltz *et al.* 2000), overall survival advantages have been seen, supporting the first-line combination approach. The trial with the highest rate of crossover also had the best survival for control arm patients (Giacchetti 1997). The UK Medical Research Council is currently running a randomised trial which includes a randomisation to '5-FU + new drug from the start' versus '5-FU until disease progression, then add new drug' in an attempt to answer this question in a structured way.

References

Barratt PL, Seymour MT, Phillips RM *et al.* (1998). The role of hMLH1, a DNA mismatch repair gene, in response to anticancer agents currently used in the treatment of colorectal cancer, in an in vitro model. *Proceedings of the American Association for Cancer Research* **39** (abstr).

Chester JD, Dent JT, Wilson G *et al.* (2000). Protracted infusional 5-fluorouracil with bolus Mitomycin in 5FU-resistant colorectal cancer. *Annals of Oncology* **11**, 235–237.

Cunningham D, Pyrhonen S, James RD *et al.* (1998). Randomised trial of irinotecan plus supportive care versus supportive care alone after fluorouracil failure for patients with metastatic colorectal cancer. *Lancet* **352**, 1413–18

De Gramont A, Bosset JF, Milan C *et al.* (1997a). Randomised trial comparing monthly low-dose leucovorin and fluorouracil bolus with bi-monthly high dose leucovorin and fluorouracil bolus plus continuous infusion for advanced colorectal cancer: a French Intergroup study. *Journal of Clinical Oncology* **15**, 808–15.

De Gramont A, Figer A, Seymour M *et al.* (2000). A randomized trial of leucovorin and 5-fluorouracil with or without oxaliplatin in advanced colorectal cancer. *Journal of Clinical Oncology* (in press).

De Gramont A, Vignoud J, Tournigand C *et al.* (1997b). Oxaliplatin with high-dose leucovorin and 5-fluorouracil 48-hour continuous infusion in pretreated metastatic colorectal cancer. *European Journal of Cancer* **33**, 214–19.

De Gramont A, Maindrault-Goebel F, Louvet C *et al.* (1999). Evaluation of oxaliplatin dose-intensity with the bimonthly 48hr leucovorin and 5-fluorouracil regimens (FOLFOX) in pretreated metastatic colorectal cancer. *Proceedings of the American Society of Clinical Oncology* **18**, 1018 (abstr).

Douillard JY, Cunningham D, Roth AD *et al.* (2000). Irinotecan combined with fluorouracil compared with fluorouracil alone as first line treatment for metastatic colorectal cancer. A multicentre randomised trial. *Lancet* **355**, 1041–7.

Fink D, Nebel S, Aebi S *et al.* (1996). The role of DNA mismatch repair in platinum drug resistance. *Cancer Research* **56**, 4881–6.

Garufi C, Brienza S, Bensmaine MA *et al.* (1995). Addition of oxaliplatin to chronomodulated 5-fluorouracil and folinic acid (FA) for reversal of acquired chemoresistance in patients with advanced colorectal cancer. *Proceedings of the American Society of Clinical Oncology* **14**, A446

Giacchetti S, Zidani R, Perpoint B *et al.* (1997). Phase III trial of 5-fluorouracil, folinic acid, with or without oxaliplatin in previously untreated patients with metastatic colorectal cancer. *Proceedings of the American Society of Clinical Oncology* **16**: 805 (abstr).

Goldie J & Coldman A (1984). The genetic origin of drug resistance in neoplasms: implications for systemic therapy. *Cancer Research* **44**, 3643–53.

Hartmann JT, Harstrick A, Daikeler T *et al.* (1998). Phase II study of continuous 120 h infusion of mitomycin C as salvage chemotherapy in patients with progressive or rapidly recurrent colorectal cancer. *Anti-Cancer Drugs* **9**, 427–31.

Levi F, Misset JL, Brienza S *et al.* (1992). A chronopharmacologic phase II clinical trial with 5-fluorouracil, folinic acid, and oxaliplatin using an ambulatory multichannel programmable pump. High antitumor effectiveness against metastatic colorectal cancer. *Cancer* **69**, 893–900.

Machover D, Diaz-Rubio E, De Gramont A *et al.* (1996). Two consecutive phase II studies of oxaliplatin for treatment of patients with advanced colorectal carcinoma who were resistant to previous treatment with fluoropyrimidines. *Annals of Oncology* **7**, 95–8.

Price T, Cunningham D, Hickish T *et al.* (1999). Phase III study of chronomodulated vs protracted venous infusional 5-fluorouracil both combined with mitomycin in first line therapy for advanced colorectal carcinoma. *Proceedings of the American Society of Clinical Oncology* **18**: 1008 (abstr).

Ratain MJ (1998). New agents for colorectal cancer: topoisomerase-I inhibitors. In *American Society of Clinical Oncology Educational Book, 34th annual meeting* (ed. MC Perry). Alexandria, VA, USA: American Society of Clinical Oncology, pp.311–15.

Ratain MJ, Goh BC, Iyer L *et al.* (1999) A phase I study of irinotecan with pharmacokinetic modulation by cyclosporin A and phenobarbital. *Proceedings of the American Society of Clinical Oncology* **18**, 777 (abstr).

Ross P, Norman A, Cunningham D *et al.* (1997). A prospective randmised trial of protracted venous infusion 5-fluorouracil with or without mitomycin C in advanced colorectal cancer. *Annals of Oncology* **8**, 995–1001.

Rothenberg ML, Hainsworth JD, Rosen L *et al.* (1998). Phase II study of irinotecan 250 mg/m^2 given every other week in previously treated colorectal cancer patients. *Proceedings of the American Society of Clinical Oncology* **17**, 1092 (abstr).

Rougier P, Bugat R, Douillard JY *et al.* (1997). Phase II study of irinotecan in the treatment of advanced colorectal cancer in chemotherapy-naive patients and patients pre-treated with fluorouracil-based chemotherapy. *Journal of Clinical Oncology* **15**, 251–60.

Rougier P, van Cutsem E, Bajetta E *et al.* (1998). Randomised trial of irinotecan versus fluorouracil by continuous infusion after fluorouracil failure in patients with metastatic colorectal cancer. *Lancet* **352**, 1407–12

Saltz L, Douillard J, Pirotta N *et al.* (2000). Combined analysis of two phase III randomized trials comparing irinotecan, fluorouracil, leucovorin vs fluorouracil alone as first-line therapy of previously untreated metastatic colorectal cancer. *Proceedings of the American Society of Clinical Oncology* **19**, 938.

Saltz L, Locker P, Pirotta N *et al.* (1999). Weekly irinotecan, leucovorin and fluorouracil is superior to daily x 5 LV/FU in patients with previously untreated metastatic colorectal cancer. *Proceedings of the American Society of Clinical Oncology* **18**, 898.

Seitz J-F, Perrier H, Giovannini M *et al.* (1998). 5-fluorouracil, high-dose folinic acid and mitomycin C combination chemotherapy in previously treated patients with advanced colorectal carcinoma. *Journal of Chemotherapy* **10**, 258–65.

Seymour M, Tabah-Fisch I, Homerin M *et al.* (1999). Quality of life in advanced colorectal cancer: a comparison of QoL during bolus plus infusional 5FU/leucovorin with or without oxaliplatin. *Proceedings of the American Society of Clinical Oncology* **18**, 901.

Tsavaris N, Ziras N, Kosmas C *et al.* (1999). Two different schedules of irinotecan administration in patients with advanced colorectal cancer relapsing after 5-fluorouracil leucovorin combination chemotherapy. Preliminary results of a randomised study. *Proceedings of the American Society of Clinical Oncology* **18**, 998 (abstr).

van Cutsem E, Rougier P, Droz JP *et al.* (1997). Clinical benefit of irinotecan in metastatic colorectal cancer resistant to 5FU. *Proceedings of the American Society of Clinical Oncology* **16**, 950 (abstract).

van Cutsem E, Bajetta E, Niederle N *et al.* (1998). A phase III multicentre randomized trial comparing CPT-11 to infusional 5FU regimen in patients with advanced colorectal cancer after 5FU failure. *Proceedings of the American Society of Clinical Oncology* **17**, 984.

Chapter 6

No treatment for the over 65s? Agreeing a definition of 'fit' and 'unfit' for chemotherapy

Kate Sumpter and Mark Hill

Introduction

Age is the greatest risk factor for the development of cancer. More than 55 per cent of malignant diseases are diagnosed in individuals over the age of 65 years. Colorectal cancer (CRC) is the second commonest cause of cancer death in the Western world. Its incidence rises with increasing age; individuals aged 80 years are three times more likely to have CRC than those aged 60 years. Currently, the majority of tumours of the colon and rectum arise in patients age 70 and over (Cancer Research Campaign 1993). Improvements in public health, nutrition and the prevention and treatment of general medical conditions have contributed to an increase in the proportion of elderly individuals in the population. The average life expectancy of a 70-year-old man is now ten years and of a 70-year-old woman, 15 years (Furner *et al.* 1997). As a result of these factors and other demographic changes, there will be a rise in the prevalence of CRC in elderly patients in the coming decades.

This chapter reviews the published data on the use of chemotherapy in elderly patients with CRC. Critical analysis of this information should inform decision making regarding which patients are deemed suitable for chemotherapy and suggest future directions for further research in this area.

Surgery for elderly patients with colorectal cancer

Elderly patients are investigated more frequently for symptoms such as anaemia, altered bowel habit and rectal bleeding than in the past. As a result, more early-stage CRCs are being identified. The operative mortality and morbidity associated with surgery for colorectal cancer have been found to be higher in the elderly in some studies (Waldron *et al.* 1986). This is attributable to the frequency of co-morbid conditions rather than to the disease itself. Improvements in peri- and post-operative care, however, have led to a dramatic improvement in these figures (Irvin 1988). Thus the great majority of patients with localised disease, regardless of their age, now receive primary surgery. The decision to operate can be taken largely independently of age but take into account co-morbid problems so that the risk:benefit ratio is defined as accurately as possible.

Adjuvant chemotherapy

The role of adjuvant chemotherapy in Dukes' C tumours of the colon and rectum following potentially curative resection is well established. Four randomised studies have shown a reduction in the risk of death by between 15 and 33 per cent (Woolmark *et al.* 1988; IMPACT 1995; O'Connell *et al.* 1997). The benefit of adjuvant chemotherapy for patients with Dukes' B tumours is less clear, with recently published data conflicting. The National Surgical Adjuvant Breast and Bowel Project (NSABP) meta-analysis showed an overall survival advantage in the order of 7 per cent for patients with Dukes' B tumours of the colon who received adjuvant chemotherapy (Mamounas *et al.* 1999). No benefit, however, was found in a similar group of patients in a sub-group analysis of the Dukes' B tumours within the IMPACT study (1999). We currently recommend adjuvant chemotherapy in the following cases:

- All medically fit patients with Dukes' C tumours;
- Patients with high risk Dukes' B tumours:
  - perforated or obstructed tumours
  - T4 tumours
  - poor differentiation on histology
  - extra-mural vascular invasion
  - mucinous differentiation.

For rectal cancer we recommend combined-modality adjuvant treatment for all Dukes' B2 and C tumours, unless the audited surgical local recurrence rates of the institution are less than 10 per cent, without routine use of radiotherapy. In this situation radiotherapy can be reserved for patients with Dukes' B3 or C3 tumours, those with positive lateral margins or those with a local recurrence.

None of the adjuvant studies mentioned thus far had an upper age limit cut-off; however, the results were not stratified according to age and therefore little information can be gained with regard to the benefits of adjuvant chemotherapy specifically in the elderly population.

There has been only one report of the use of adjuvant chemotherapy stratified according to age (Brower *et al.* 1993). In this study the records of 111 patients treated with post-operative chemotherapy after curative surgery were reviewed, patients were categorised into those aged under 70 years, those aged 70–74 and those aged 75 and over. The average early-dose intensity for patients over 75 was lower than the other two age groups and whether the lower doses given to the elderly achieve the same results as those administered to the young remains questionable. The concern that older patients have greater toxicity with chemotherapy has led to caution in recommendations regarding adjuvant chemotherapy in the over-75s.

A study of adjuvant chemotherapy from the Royal Marsden Hospital analysed the toxicity of systemic protracted venous infusion (PVI) 5-fluorouracil (5-FU) 300 mg/m^2 daily and of bolus injections of 5-FU and folinic acid according to the NCCTG/Mayo regimen (Popescu *et al.* 1999). The data for elderly patients (defined as those over 70 years of age) were compared to data for the younger population. In total 543 patients received either PVI 5-FU or bolus 5-FU. Of these, 422 were less than 70 years of age (214 received bolus, 208 PVI 5-FU) and 121 were aged over 70 (72 bolus, 49 PVI 5-FU). The toxicity data for both treatments were analysed, and the only significant difference in toxicity noted between the two age groups was in the incidence of stomatitis, which was significantly higher in the age group over 70 years (p=0.02). This difference was seen only in the elderly patients receiving the bolus NCCTG regime. The survival data are not yet mature and await analysis.

Over recent decades, life expectancy has improved significantly. With these improvements, particularly in a disease such as colorectal cancer in which recurrent disease occurs predominantly within the first three years of primary surgery, one can see potential benefit for elderly patients being treated in the adjuvant setting. On this basis, the authors recommend that elderly patients should be considered for adjuvant chemotherapy using similar criteria to younger patients.

Palliative therapy

The benefits of palliative 5-FU-based chemotherapy have been confirmed in three randomised studies, comparing the use of either intravenous or hepatic artery infusion chemotherapy with best supportive care only (The Nordic Gastrointestinal Tumor Adjuvant Therapy Group 1992; Scheithauer *et al.* 1993; Allen-Mersh *et al.* 1994). A further study by Baretta *et al.* (1994) performed a sub-group randomisation for elderly patients (aged 70 years of age and over). They were randomised between receiving leucovorin 240 mg/m^2 IV bolus + 5-FU and 180 mg/m^2 IV bolus repeated weekly for six months or until disease progression or to supportive care only. The results of this study showed a statistically significant overall survival benefit (P<0.002) for chemotherapy over supportive care. The authors concluded that elderly patients as well as younger patients benefited from palliative weekly 5-FU + leucovorin.

However, there are no other prospective randomised control trials which deal specifically with chemotherapy for elderly patients with CRC. At the Royal Marsden Hospital, a recently published analysis used information from a prospective database to analyse the chemotherapy toxicity, response and survival in elderly patients treated with either 5-FU or raltitrexed for metastatic colorectal cancer (Popescu *et al.* 1999). The elderly group was compared with data for the younger patient population. A total of 844 patients were treated within a locally advanced or metastatic disease protocol, 658 of these were under 70 years of age and 186 were 70 and over. The median age for these two groups was 58 years and 73 years, respectively. The chemotherapy regimes employed were predominantly PVI 5-FU (300 mg/m^2 per day continuous infusion), PVI 5-FU + mitomycin-C 7-10 mg/m^2 six weekly, PVI 5-FU + interferon – α, raltitrexed and bolus 5-FU/leucovorin, according to the NCCTG regime. The age distribution was well balanced between these treatments. The toxicity analysis revealed no significant difference in the numbers experiencing overall or severe toxicity between patients under or over 70 years of age. The response rates to first-line metastatic chemotherapy were 24 per cent in patients aged 70 or older compared to 29 per cent in younger patients (p=0.19). There was no difference in the overall failure-free survival between these two groups (164 versus 169 days, respectively) or the one-year failure free survival (18 versus 19 per cent, respectively). There was, however, a shorter median overall survival in the elderly group (292 versus 350 days, p=0.04), but this included non-cancer-related deaths (see Table 6.1). This study suggests that chemotherapy in elderly patients with colorectal cancer is in fact well tolerated and has similar palliative benefits regarding response rates and failure-free survival to chemotherapy in younger patients. The patients included in this study were performance status 0–2 and careful selection of patients, rather than age, is probably the most important factor when considering who would be a suitable candidate for chemotherapy.

Table 6.1 Response rates and survival to palliative chemotherapy based on age

	<70 years	>70 years	P
Response rate	29%	24%	0.19
FFS	169 days	164 days	0.862
Overall survival	350 days	292 days	0.04

Source: Popescu *et al.* (1999)

Further work from the National Institute for Cancer Research in Italy has been published using data from two consecutive trials, comparing the results of toxicity and efficacy of treatment in patients 65 years of age and older compared with those under 65 years (Chiara *et al.* 1998): 215 patients were included, of whom 82 by their criteria were classified as elderly. The median age of this elderly population was 70 years and the median performance status was 1. All patients received one of the following 5-FU based regimens:

- weekly 5-FU 600 mg/m^2 IV bolus;
- same 5-FU + leucovorin 500 mg/m^2 weekly;
- weekly 5-FU 260 mg/m^2 24-hour continuous infusion + leucovorin 100 mg/m^2 four-hour IV infusion and subsequently orally for five doses.

The main toxicities observed in this study were diarrhoea, stomatitis and hand-foot syndrome. There were no significant differences in toxicity between patients under or over 65 years of age. The median dose intensity was no different between the two groups. The overall objective response rate was 18 per cent in the elderly patients compared with 23 per cent in patients under 65 years of age. This study again confirms that advanced age is not a contraindication to the use of chemotherapy, particularly 5-FU-based regimes.

In addition to these two studies, Begg & Carbone (1993) have reported on the Eastern and Cooperative Oncology Group (ECOG) experience of toxicity and survival in 19 trials for advanced cancer, including colorectal cancer. They reviewed 1,210 cases, of which 174 were aged over 70 years. There was no difference in toxicity rates across the age cut-off. A similarly supportive study performed by Cascinu *et al.* (1996) again did not find any differences in toxicity or response rates in a matched controlled case study of 120 patients with advanced cancers at six different sites, including colorectal cancer, using an age cut-off at 70 years.

Stein *et al.* (1995) performed an analysis on data from a multi-institutional prospective randomised phase III trial of 5-FU-based chemotherapy in metastatic colorectal cancer. There was no upper age limit and the study population was divided into younger (aged up to 70 years), and older (aged 70 years and over) groups. There were four treatment arms:

- 5-FU 500 mg/m^2 IV bolus day 1–5 every 28 days;
- 5-FU 600 mg/m^2 IV bolus + leucovorin 500 mg/m^2 over two hours weekly times six every eight weeks;
- 5-FU 600 mg/m^2 IV bolus + leucovorin 25 mg/m^2 weekly times six every eight weeks;
- 5-FU 1,000 mg/m^2 IV bolus + 25 mg/m^2 of leucovorin every three weeks.

This fourth arm was abandoned because of a poor response rate and was not included in the analysis. A total of 331 patients were treated in one of the three remaining arms and data were available for toxicity analysis. The majority (264) of these were under 70 years of age but 67 were over 70. Significant associations were found on univariate analysis between age and severe toxicity ($p<0.001$), leucopenia ($p<0.005$), diarrhoea ($p=0.01$), vomiting ($p=0.01$) and death ($p=0.01$). Women showed a greater incidence of toxicity, with significant differences observed in any severe toxicity ($p<0.0001$), leucopenia ($p<0.0005$), infection ($p<0.005$), diarrhoea ($p<0.01$), multi-organ system toxicity ($p=0.01$) and vomiting ($p=0.03$). Interestingly, there was no statistically significant association between performance status and toxicity. Logistic regression confirmed age to be a highly significant independent predictor of severe toxicity, as was sex.

There are discrepancies, therefore, in the results of the few trials that have been performed in elderly patients with CRC evaluating the benefits and toxicity of palliative chemotherapy. These are perhaps best explained by the knowledge that the toxicity of 5-FU is schedule-dependent. Small differences in dosage or modulation of 5-FU can lead to large changes in the toxicity profile. The Meta-Analysis Group in Cancer study (1998), comparing continuous infusion with bolus administration of 5-FU, showed higher tumour response rate, overall survival and lower severe toxicity (except plantar palmar erythema) in patients with advanced colorectal cancer receiving continuous infusion 5-FU. Treatment regimes with lower toxicity and an easier schedule of administration would of course be of benefit to the entire patient population but perhaps more so to the elderly. Oral fluoropyrimidines have for these reasons been developed: however, they are not without toxicity and prior to their widespread use in the elderly, their safety and efficacy needs to be established.

There have been two reports of phase II studies using oral fluoropyrimidines; the first utilised UFT, which contains 1-(2-tetrahydrofuryl)-5-fluorouracil (tegafur) and uracil in a molar ratio 1:4 (Feliu *et al.* 1997). Tegafur is converted to 5-FU by the enzyme thymidine phosphorylase, and uracil inhibits the catabolism of 5-FU by competing with the patient's hepatic dihydropyrimidine dehydrogenase (DPD). Thirty-eight patients aged over 70 with previously untreated advanced colorectal cancer and performance status 0–2 were included in the study. Treatment consisted of leucovorin 500 mg/m^2 IV over two hours on day 1 + UFT 390 mg/m^2 (in two divided doses) per day on days 1–14 and oral leucovorin 15 mg bd on days 2–14. Treatment cycles were repeated every 28 days. The median number of treatment cycles received was seven per patient. The overall response rate was 29 per cent. Toxicities were mild and consisted of 10 per cent grade 3–4 diarrhoea; one patient experienced grade 3–4 nausea and vomiting; and one patient experienced grade 3–4 mucositis. Of interest, grade 3–4 toxicity was more frequent among women than men (38 versus 4 per cent, $p<0.05$). The study demonstrated that the combination of UFT and leucovorin was active and well tolerated in older patients, but close monitoring of elderly women would be warranted in view of their increased risk of toxicity.

The second study of oral agents in the elderly used doxifluridine, which is activated to 5-FU by uridine phosphorylase (an enzyme with high levels of expression in malignant cells) (Falcone *et al.* 1994). It involved 43 patients aged 69–83 years, with a median age of 74 and performance status 0–2. All had previously untreated metastatic colorectal cancer. Doxifluridine was given orally at an initial daily dose of 2,250 mg for four consecutive days every week. Dose reduction was employed if grade 2 or more toxicity occurred. Grade 3–4 toxicity was uncommon, with diarrhoea the most frequent at 17 per cent. The overall response rate was 14 per cent, which is similar to that seen with intravenous unmodulated fluoropyrimidines. Studies are ongoing to improve the clinical activity of doxifluridine by combining it with oral folinic acid.

There are a number of recognised prognostic factors in metastatic colorectal cancer: performance status, tumour differentiation, serum carcinoembryonic antigen (CEA) levels, original Dukes' stage, serum lactate dehydrogenase (LDH), tumour size and primary tumour location. Edler *et al.* (1986) conducted a multivariate analysis on data from the Chemotherapy of Gastrointestinal Tumours Study Group, who performed a number of clinical trials of chemotherapy in metastatic colorectal cancer. The aim of the analysis was to extract the most significant factors predicting for survival. All 139 patients received chemotherapy within the context of clinical trials, and their records were examined retrospectively. The regimens were all fluoropyrimidine-based, some involving combinations with drugs such as mitomycin C and BCNU. Performance status was classified according to the Swiss oncology group (SAKK) system, which is similar to the ECOG: PS 0 normal activity; PS 1 patient able to live independently with tolerable tumour manifestations; PS 2 patient has disabling tumour manifestations but is in bed for less than 50 per cent of the time; PS 3 patient is in bed for more than 50 per cent of the time; PS 4 patient is very sick and bedridden. Thrity-three characteristics were considered for their prognostic significance. On univariate analysis the following factors were strong indicators of survival (all $p<0.01$): performance status, size of primary tumour, loss of weight, alkaline phosphatase, albumin, white blood count, haemoglobin and blood sedimentation rate. Of these, performance status exhibited the highest level of significance. Patients with PS 1 or 2 showed a three to five times increased risk of death than those with PS 0; those with PS 3 or 4 had a 20-time greater risk of death. It can be seen from the above that performance status is a far more useful indicator of the likely benefit from chemotherapy than is age.

Conclusions

Despite the fact that colorectal cancer is predominantly a disease of the elderly, there is a paucity of randomised prospective data where the use of chemotherapy in elderly patients is specifically studied. While many trials do not have an age cut-off, rarely are stratifications included to account for age.

Elderly patients can have increased toxicity with chemotherapy compared to their younger counterparts but this is in part due to co-morbid conditions. This highlights the importance of treatment with minimal toxicity such as systemic protracted venous infusion 5-FU.

The criteria by which patients are deemed to be fit for chemotherapy should be based on factors known to influence outcome, the most important of which is performance status. We would not recommend palliative chemotherapy for patients with PS 3 or 4, regardless of their age.

Placing an age cut-off for treatment is entirely arbitrary since the biological age of patients can often be considerably different from the chronological age. Elderly patients should be informed of treatment options in the same way as younger individuals. The optimal approach to treatment of any patient remains the provision of maintained or improved quality of life for the maximum duration of time whilst balancing these benefits against the known risks of therapy.

References

Allen-Mersh TG *et al.* (1994) Quality of life and survival with continuous hepatic-artery floxuridine infusion for colorectal liver metastasis. *Lancet* **344**, 1255–60.

Begg CB *et al.* (1983). The experience of the Eastern Cooperative Oncology Group. *Cancer* **52**, 1986–92.

Beretta G *et al.* (1994). Fluorouracil + folates (FUFO) as standard treatment for advanced/metastatic gastrointestinal carcinomas (AGC). *Annals of Oncology* **5** (suppl.8), 239.

Brower M *et al.* (1993). Adjuvant chemotherapy for colorectal cancer in the elderly: population-based experience. *Proceedings of the American Society of Clinical Oncology* **12**, 195.

Cancer Research Campaign (1993). *Cancer of the Large Bowel.* London: Cancer Research Campaign.

Cascinu S *et al.* (1996) Toxicity and therapeutic response to chemotherapy in patients aged 70 years or older with advanced cancer. *American Journal of Clinical Oncology* **19**, 371–4.

Chiara S *et al.* (1998). Advanced colorectal cancer ion the elderly: results of consecutive trials with 5-fluorouracil-based chemotherapy. *Cancer Chemother Pharmacol* **42**, 336–40.

Edler L *et al.* (1986). Prognostic factors of advanced colorectal cancer patients. *European Journal of Clinical Oncology* **22**,1231–7.

Falcone A *et al.* (1994). Oral doxifluridine in elderly patients with metastatic colorectal cancer: a multicenter phase II study. *Annals of Oncology* **5,** 760–2.

Feliu J *et al.* (1997). Uracil and tegafur modulated with leucovorin. An effective regimen with low toxicity for the treatment of colorectal carcinoma in the elderly. *Cancer* **79**, 1884–9.

Furner SE *et al.* (1997). Epidemiology and aging. In *Geriatric Medicine* 3rd edn (ed. CK Cassel *et al.*), pp.37–43. Springer, New York (USA).

[IMPACT] International Multi-centre Pooled Analysis of Colon Cancer Trial (IMPACT) investigators (1995). Efficacy of adjuvant fluorouracil and folinic acid in colon cancer. *Lancet* **354**, 939–44.

[IMPACT] International Multicentre Pooled Analysis of B2 Colon Cancer Trials (IMPACT B2) Investigators (1999). Efficacy of adjuvant fluorouracil and folinic acid in B2 colon cancer. *Journal of Clinical Oncology* **17**, 1356–63.

Irvin TT (1988). Prognosis of Colorectal Cancer in the elderly. *British Journal of Surgery* **5**, 419–21.

Mamounas E *et al.* (1999). Comparative efficacy of adjuvant chemotherapy in patients with Dukes' B versus Dukes' C colon cancer: results from four National Surgical Adjuvant Breast and Bowel Project Adjuvant Studies (C-01, C-02, C-03, and C-04). *Journal of Clinical Oncology* **17**, 1349–55.

The Meta-Analysis Group in Cancer (1998). Efficacy of intravenous continuous infusion of fluoruracil compared with bolus administration in advanced colorectal cancer. *Journal of Clinical Oncology* **16**, 301–8.

Moertel C *et al.* (1990). Levamisole and fluorouracil for adjuvant therapy of resected colon carcinoma. *New England Journal of Medicine* **322**, 352–8.

The Nordic Gastrointestinal Tumor Adjuvant Therapy Group (1992). Expectancy or primary chemotherapy in patients with advanced asymptomatic colorectal cancer: a randomised trial, *Journal of Clinical Oncology* **10**, 904–11.

O'Connell M *et al.* (1997). Controlled trial of fluorouracil and low dose of leucovorin given for six months as post-operative adjuvant therapy for colon cancer. *Journal of Clinical Oncology* **15**, 246–50.

Popescu R *et al.* (1999). Adjuvant or palliative chemotherapy for colorectal cancer in patients seventy years or older. *Journal of Clinical Oncology* (in press).

Scheithauer W *et al.* (1993). Randomised comparison of combination chemotherapy plus supportive care alone in patients with metastatic colorectal cancer. *British Medical Journal* **306**, 752–5.

Stein B *et al.* (1995). Age and sex are independent predictors of 5-fluorouracil toxicity. Analysis of a large scale phase III trial. *Cancer* **75**, 11–17.

Waldron RP *et al.* (1986). Emergency presentation and mortality from colorectal cancer in the elderly. *British Journal of Surgery* **73**, 214–16.

Wolmark N *et al.* (1988). Post-operative adjuvant chemotherapy or BCG for colon cancer colon results from NSABP protocol C-01. *Journal of the National Cancer Institute* **80**, 30–36.

PART 3

Focus on rectal cancer

Evaluation of MRI as an effective means of pre-operative staging in rectal cancer

Gina Brown

Introduction

In patients with rectal cancer, local recurrence is an important cause of morbidity and mortality. The results of surgery for removal of local recurrences are uniformly poor, and the symptoms of intractable pelvic pain from local recurrence are extremely difficult to palliate (Frykholm *et al.* 1995*)*. Thus current treatment strategies are aimed at reducing the local recurrence rate. The primary surgical procedure is of crucial importance in achieving local cure (Heald *et al.* 1982, 1986, 1998); good lateral clearance and the use of total mesorectal excision techniques have improved recurrence rates. However, despite this, up to 25 per cent of rectal resection specimens examined in 1994 had inadequate margins (Adam *et al.* 1994).

Current treatment strategies and the relevance of pre-operative imaging

A number of controlled trials have shown a reduction in local recurrence rates in patients treated with pre-operative radiotherapy (Gerard *et al.* 1988; Cedermark *et al.* 1990, 1994, 1995; Marsh *et al.* 1994; Pahlman & Glimelius 1995). The current multimodality approach for treatment of patients with rectal cancer depends on the pre-operative identification of specific surgical risk groups (Baigrie & Berry 1994). Studies demonstrating the benefit of pre-operative neoadjuvant therapy and adjuvant radiotherapy need to be balanced against the inevitable cost, short and long-term morbidity and survival gain compared with optimised conventional surgical therapy. It seems likely that patient selection will play an important role in determining which patients should undergo intensive pre-operative chemoradiation schedules.

It has been advocated that short-course pre-operative radiotherapy is given to patients at risk of local failure; that is, patients with primarily resectable tumours but in whom there is tumour penetration through the bowel wall or lymph node involvement (Baigrie & Berry 1994; Pahlman & Glimelius 1999). This treatment is not, however, appropriate for patients with locally extensive tumours or patients with generalised disease (Pahlman & Glimelius 1999), and such patients may benefit from intensive pre-operative chemoradiation in an attempt to downstage tumour and render the tumour operable for cure (Minsky *et al.* 1997; Marsh *et al.* 1996). Conversely, patients with tumour confined to the bowel wall without evidence of lymph node involvement who are likely to be cured by surgery alone could be excluded from receiving potentially harmful pre-operative therapy (Dahlberg *et al.* 1998). These differences in treatment strategies based on pre-operative multimodality treatment thus require an accurate pre-operative staging method.

Accurate pre-operative staging

Accurate spatial depiction of the anatomical disposition of the primary rectal tumour and associated deposits is essential to developing an optimised surgical approach in rectal cancer surgery. The relationship of the tumour to the mesorectal fascia and adjacent organs will determine whether a conventional mesorectal excision may be performed or a more extended radical approach is needed in order to achieve negative circumferential margins (Yasutomi *et al.* 1997; Verschueren *et al.* 1998). The accurate depiction of the lower edge of tumour in relation to the anal sphincter complex will influence the decision whether sphincter-saving surgery is possible, or whether pre-operative chemoradiation should be offered in order to facilitate sphincter-saving surgery (Janjan *et al.* 1999; Vauthey *et al.* 1999). Further potential benefits of accurate pre-operative staging include a reduction in the number of open and close laparotomies and pre-operative examinations under anaesthesia for tumours that cannot be assessed clinically.

Pre-operative adjuvant and neoadjuvant therapy issues

In assessing, comparing and planning chemoradiation regimes there is a need for reliable and accurate delineation of the primary tumour. This is not only important for patient selection but also to obtain an objective measure of the extent of tumour at the outset so that the true extent of downstaging may be assessed by comparing final histopathology with pre-treatment imaging (Wheeler *et al.* 1999). Thus, a quantifiable assessment of the efficacy of particular chemoradiation treatment protocols may be achieved.

Important prognostic factors that should be assessed by imaging

Depth of penetration through the bowel wall

Pelvic recurrence in rectal cancer appears to be related to the inability to obtain wide circumferential margins even though proximal and distal resection margins may be adequate (Adam *et al.* 1994). Such local recurrences are associated with survival rates of only 6 per cent. Dukes' seminal paper (1932) highlighted the importance of the extent of extramural spread in the prediction of local recurrence as well as survival. Survival figures for Dukes' B cases were 89.7 per cent for slight spread, 80 per cent for moderate spread and 57 per cent for extensive spread. This measurement is taken from the outer edge of the longitudinal muscle layer.

Another important feature is that, once spread beyond the bowel wall occurs, the incidence of lymph node invasion rises from 14.2 per cent in tumours confined to the bowel wall to 43.2 per cent in tumours extending beyond the bowel wall. Regardless of lymph node status, it has been shown by the St Marks' group that survival was 97 per cent in those tumours with no spread beyond the bowel wall (Jass 1995; Jass *et al.* 1986, 1987).

Work by Harrison *et al.* (1994) also showed that the extent of tumour spread beyond the muscularis propria externa was an important and independent prognostic factor. Patients with widely invasive tumours had a significantly worse survival than patients with slight or moderate extramural spread. Studies evaluating patients with local recurrence have shown that tumour penetration through the bowel wall is significantly related to survival (Lindmark *et al.* 1994). Thus patients with tumour penetration through the bowel wall receive a five-day course of high-dose pre-operative radiotherapy, with immediate surgery upon completion of radiotherapy. For patients with extensive tumour penetration in whom local resection is unlikely to result in circumferential margins clear of tumour, a longer course of radiotherapy is advocated (Baigrie & Berry 1994). This has been shown to improve local control; in addition, some of these patients may be rendered operable by long-course radiotherapy owing to radiation induced tumour downstaging (Pahlman & Glimelius 1995).

Distance of tumour from anorectal junction

A low anterior resection is the standard procedure for carcinoma of the upper rectum. For carcinoma of the mid- and lower rectum, precise knowledge of the distal extent of tumour will determine the surgical choice between an abdominoperineal resection and a sphincter-preserving anterior resection. This knowledge is normally gained by digital rectal examination but this is limited to an assessment of the palpable intraluminal tumour. The extraluminal component of the tumour and its distance from the anorectal junction cannot therefore be assessed by digital rectal examination. Knowledge of the precise site of the tumour is also important in pre-operative radiotherapy planning. Pre-operative staging must, therefore, accurately identify the distal extent of tumour.

Spread beyond the peritoneal membrane

Local peritoneal involvement is of prognostic influence in rectal cancer and may predict some cases of local recurrence after surgery for upper and middle rectal cancer. Local peritoneal involvement was detected in 25.8 per cent (54/209) of cases (Shepherd *et al.* 1995). Local peritoneal involvement is associated with considerable prognostic disadvantage in all cases. This is a particular problem in upper rectal cancers.

Lymph node staging

The existence of large tumour nodules and metastatic lymph nodes is closely correlated with the presence of microscopic cancer and a poor prognostic subgroup (Ueno *et al.* 1998). The importance of adequate clearance in such patients is highlighted (Hida *et al.* 1997), but Ueno *et al.* suggest that palpation of tumour nodules at the time of surgery and fresh frozen biopsy assessment is a means of identifying such patients. Clearly, the pre-operative identification of these would enable patient selection for additional pre-operative therapy.

Venous spread

Spread into thick-walled extramural veins carries a very poor prognosis (Talbot *et al.* 1981). The corrected five-year survival for Dukes' stage C patients with invasion of thick-walled veins was only 8 per cent. Invasion of extramural veins was associated with a low five-year survival rate of 33 per cent. In the model using step-wise selection of prognostic indicators, extramural venous invasion retained independent prognostic significance (Harrison *et al.* 1994).

Current methods of local staging in rectal cancer

Digital rectal examination

Digital rectal examination (DRE) remains the current widely used mode of pre-operative patient treatment selection for pre-operative therapy in the UK. The technique relies on the ability of the examiner to assess the fixity of a low rectal tumour. A freely mobile tumour is said to represent tumour confined to the bowel wall and therefore treatable by optimised surgery alone. Tethered tumours are said to represent tumours with invasion into perirectal tissues and are thus suitable for optimised surgery with possible pre-operative radiotherapy. Fixed tumours are those that are considered fixed to adjacent organs and therefore surgically unresectable for cure. This method of staging was shown to have accuracy in 80 per cent of cases, in one series, and fixity was found to be associated with a poorer prognosis; however, in a study by Durdey & Williams (1984), 26 per cent of tumours were tethered due to perirectal inflammation only. Patients who cannot be assessed by endoluminal ultrasound are currently only evaluated by DRE, which may need to be performed under general anaesthesia for mid/upper rectal tumours. Staging by DRE is limited to an assessment of fixity or tethering of the tumour in an attempt to identify locally invasive tumours for radical radiotherapy. DRE has not been shown to be an accurate method of staging rectal tumours (Kusonoki *et al.* 1994).

Table 7.1 Local staging by DRE – advantages and disadvantages

Advantages	Disadvantages
❏ Inexpensive	❏ Costly for low, bulky or painful tumours as DRE needs to be performed under general anaesthesia
❏ Accuracy of up to 80 per cent in experienced observers	❏ 20–30 per cent of tumours are too high or impalpable
	❏ Overstaging and understaging due to examiner's inexperience, apparent fixity due to peritumoral inflammation, fibrosis or bulky intraluminal tumours within small pelvis
	❏ Inability to relate tumour to mesorectal fascia
	❏ Inability to detect higher tumour deposits within the mesorectum
	❏ Cannot identify patients with extramural venous invasion or peritoneal invasion

Endoluminal ultrasound

Accuracy as high as 90 per cent have been documented in staging rectal cancer by endoluminal ultrasound (EUS) (Beynon 1994; Massari *et al.* 1998; Adams *et al.* 1999; Maldjian *et al.* 2000). However, these studies have evaluated selected patients – excluding patients with clinically fixed tumours, tumours of the upper rectum and patients with bulky or stenosing tumours. Thus, up to 20 per cent of patients presenting with rectal cancer cannot be evaluated by endorectal ultrasound (Lindmark *et al.* 1992). Many of these bulky/stricturing tumours are likely to be T3/T4 and the very cases that need to be accurately. Furthermore, when tumour penetrates through the bowel wall, contrast between bowel wall and perirectal fat may be lost and assessment of the depth of tumour penetration may be inaccurate (Lindmark *et al.* 1992). The limitations of EUS include its small field of view and inability to stage high, stricturing or painful tumours. Furthermore, tumours with a bulky intraluminal projection can only be examined by placing the probe tangential rather than perpendicular to the tumour, resulting in difficulties in interpretation of the depth of tumour invasion (Akasu *et al.* 1997) A further limitation is the inability to allow peritumoural fibrosis to be distinguished from tumour (Maier *et al.* 1997). The small field of view prevents demonstration of the relationship of the tumour to the mesorectal fascia, which is the plane through which total mesorectal excision takes place (Akasu *et al.* 1997).

Computed tomography (CT) staging in rectal cancer

The usefulness of computed tomography (CT) in the staging of rectal cancer has been disappointing (Mehta *et al.* 1994; Zerhouni *et al.* 1996; Kim *et al.* 1999). The main problems relate to the inability of this modality to visualise the layers of

Table 7.2 Local staging by endoluminal ultrasound – advantages and disadvantages

Advantages	Disadvantages
❏ Inexpensive	❏ Unsuitable for assessment of bulky or painful tumours
❏ Accuracy of up to 80 per cent in experienced observers	❏ 20–30 per cent of tumours are too high or impalpable
	❏ Overstaging and understaging due to observer inexperience, overstaging due to peritumoral inflammation, fibrosis
	❏ Inability to relate tumour to mesorectal fascia
	❏ Inability to detect higher tumour deposits within the mesorectum
	❏ Cannot identify patients with extramural venous invasion or peritoneal invasion

the bowel wall. The main criterion for identification of tumour is thickening but this is non-specific and may be due to fibrosis, inflammation or oblique sectioning through the tumour on CT, which employs transverse sectioning through the pelvis rather than axial to the tumour. Importantly, the longitudinal muscle layer is irregular and this may account for overstaging as well as 'spiculation' used as a criterion for local perirectal invasion which in fact is due to desmoplastic reaction and not tumour infiltration (Thoeni *et al.* 1981). Inability to depict the mesorectal fascia, except in extensive disease (Grabbe *et al.* 1983) that has invaded and thickened it, makes this an ineffective technique when planning the margins for resection. The inaccuracy of CT in lymph node detection also relates to the use of size criteria which can result in both overstaging of nodes and understaging of normal-sized nodes. Other problems relate to inability to depict the anal sphincter in relation to tumour, resulting in inability to predict anal sphincter invasion. Despite initial enthusiasm for the technique, CT is not recommended for the local staging of rectal tumours, and its inaccuracy rules it out as a means of detecting or demonstrating response to pre-operative therapy, as it will fail to distinguish between residual tumour and fibrosis (Zerhouni *et al.* 1996; Kim *et al.* 1999).

Magnetic resonance imaging

A number of studies have evaluated magnetic resonance imaging (MRI) in the staging of rectal cancer. These studies, however, employed conventional spin-echo imaging, used large fields of view and thick slices, obtaining lower resolution scans. The images produced were thus unable to depict the layers of the rectal wall (Kusunoki *et al.* 1994; Mcnicholas *et al.* 1994; Zerhouni *et al.* 1996). Overstaging in patients occurred as a result of the inability to depict a clear line of cleavage between tumour and adjacent structures (Mcnicholas *et al.* 1994; Thaler *et al.* 1994). A study evaluating endorectal MRI was able to demonstrate the layers using T2-weighted fast

Table 7.3 Local staging of rectal cancer by CT – advantages and disadvantages

Advantages	Disadvantages
❏ Suitable for assessment of bulky or painful tumours	❏ Overstaging due to inability to distinguish peritumoral inflammation and fibrosis
❏ Locally advanced tumours accurately staged	❏ Overestimation of tumour depth due to imaging rectal wall obliquely
	❏ Poor contrast between rectal wall and tumour
	❏ Inability to depict the mesorectal fascia or peritoneal reflection
	❏ Inability to identify or characterise tumour deposits within the mesorectum
	❏ Cannot identify anal sphincter complex as a separate structure
	❏ Cannot identify patients with extramural venous invasion or peritoneal invasion

spin-echo (FSE) imaging (Schnall & Kressel 1994). However, it was recognised that the use of such a coil created problems related to mucosal distortion by the balloon effectively obliterating the submucosa–muscle interface. Another problem was the inability to produce a circumferential image of the rectum due to the offset nature of the coil. The main limitation of the endorectal coil is that it cannot be employed to assess patients with bulky or stricturing tumours, in whom the coil cannot be passed; thus patients not assessable by EUS because of stricturing would also be unsuitable for endorectal MRI assessment.

Thin-slice, high-resolution MRI

Thin-slice, high-resolution MRI uses thin 3 mm, small field of view, high image matrix imaging (Table 7.4). Using this scanning technique and a surface pelvic coil rather than an endorectal coil, a similar in-plane resolution could be achieved as that obtained with an endorectal coil (0.6 x 0.6 mm). The potential advantages of this technique include the ability to evaluate all patients since an invasive endorectal coil is not employed. A pilot study evaluating high-resolution MRI of the pelvis established reporting criteria by detailed comparison of thin-slice MRI with histology (Brown *et al.* 1996): a total of 133 in vivo and specimen image slice were staged prospectively (TNM staging) and compared with the corresponding histopathological slice stage. The agreement for T-stage between individual MRI slices and the corresponding histopathological slices was 88 per cent (k=0.84). The images obtained thus depicted all layers of the rectal wall. No patient preparation was necessary for MRI scanning of the rectum. An advantage of using this technique is the ability to image a relatively large area of the perirectal tissue. On the FSE T2-weighted images perirectal fat is of higher signal than tumour, allowing clear visualisation of tumour extension into fat.

Table 7.4 Thin slice MRI technique

Axial and sagittal T2-weighted fast-spin echo acquisitions of the anatomical pelvis:
– 24 cm field of view
– 5 mm contiguous slice thickness
– TR>2500 ms, <6000 ms, TE 85 ms
– 512 x 256 matrix
– echo train length of 8 and 2 acquisitions

These scans will be used to plan high-resolution axial scans through the rectal tumour and adjacent pararectal tissues:
– 16 cm field of view
– 3 mm slice thickness, no interslice gap
– TR >2500 ms,<6000 ms, TE 85 ms
– 256 x 256 matrix
– echo train length of 8 and 4 acquisitions.
– the mean time taken to complete each patient examination in a pilot study was 40 minutes (range 35–65 minutes)

Normal anatomy as depicted by high resolution MRI

The bowel wall layers comprise the mucosal layer as a fine low signal intensity line with the thicker higher signal submucosal layer lying beneath this. The muscularis propria can sometimes be depicted as two distinct layers – the inner circular layer and the outer longitudinal layer. The outer muscle layer has an irregular corrugated appearance and there are frequently interruptions within this layer due to vessels entering the rectal wall. The perirectal fat appears as high signal surrounding the low signal of the muscularis propria (Brown *et al.* 1999).

The mesorectal fascia is seen as a fine low signal layer enveloping the perirectal fat and rectum; it is this layer that defines the surgical excision plane in total mesorectal excision surgery.

The peritoneal reflection lies on the surface of the bladder and then attaches itself to the anterior aspect of the rectal wall. This is consistently seen on the sagittal T2 weighted scans and so the relationship of the tumour to the peritoneal reflection attachment may be determined.

Tumour morphology

The criteria for image interpretation are summarised in Table 7.5 (Brown *et al.* 1999). It is important to stress that MR diagnosis of T3 lesions is based on the presence of tumour signal extending into perirectal fat with a broad-based bulging configuration (Figure 7.1), and in continuity with the intramural portion of the tumour. Irregularity and disruption of the outer longitudinal muscle in themselves do not signify T3 tumour, as interruptions of the outer contour of the muscle coat of the

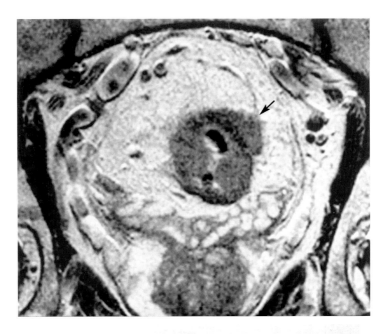

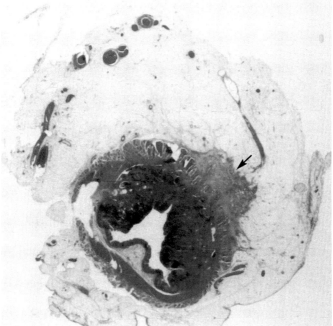

Figure 7.1 Axial T2 weighted high-resolution image and corresponding wholemount histopathology section depicting a semi-annular tumour of the mid-rectum. The tumour is centred on the posterior wall of the rectum and extends into perirectal fat posterolaterally with a characteristic broad-based pushing margin (arrow)

Table 7.5 MRI reporting criteria for T and N staging of rectal carcinoma

T1 lesion	A low signal mass demonstrated within the bright mucosal/ submucosal layer but with preservation of the muscularis propria layer
T2 lesion	A low signal mass demonstrated within the submucosal layer causing loss of the interface between the submucosa and muscularis propria
T3 lesion	Tumour is of higher signal intensity than muscle. Breach of the outer rectal longitudinal muscle layer with broad based/nodular extension of the tumour signal into the perirectal fat
T4 lesion	Extension of tumour signal intensity into adjacent structures or extension through peritoneal reflection in high anterior rectal tumours
Nodal involvement	Presence of involved perirectal lymph nodes – tumour signal/nodes with irregular or ill-defined contour

rectum occur normally as a result of small vessels penetrating the wall. Furthermore, the longitudinal muscle layer itself often has an irregular corrugated appearance in the absence of tumour. We have observed that, having penetrated the bowel wall, these tumours could spread over a large distance above or below the intraluminal portion of the tumour in the perirectal fat. This degree of spread would not be appreciated by direct visualisation sigmoidoscopy and would be difficult using EUS owing to its inherent small field of view. This MRI technique therefore not only has the potential for assessing all patients rather than a subgroup, but it also provides more information relevant to pre-operative treatment planning than other staging methods.

Tumours with gross pushing margins were most often associated with extensive nodal involvement and vascular invasion. We believe the finding on MRI of gross extramural spread is correlated with a distinct sub-group of patients with poor prognosis. Although there were undoubted cases of T2 and minimal T3 tumours in our series with nodal involvement, the nodal involvement was such that only one or two small (<5 mm) nodes were involved. This was in contrast with the more extensive and larger nodal deposits noted in the cases with gross extramural spread. The difference in these two groups is known from studies that have looked at the differing survivals of the Astler Collins' stage C1 compared with stage C2 tumours (Chung *et al.* 1983). Few pathological studies have compared extramural spread with prognosis but Cawthorn *et al.* (1990) have shown that extramural spread is an independent prognostic predictor of poor outcome. It is possible that pre-operative detection of this feature would allow appropriate selection of patients for neoadjuvant therapy. The MR features of mucinous tumours were distinctive as these had very high signal as opposed to the low/intermediate signal intensity of all other rectal tumours. Pre-operative biopsy of these tumours did not always reveal their mucinous nature. Spiculation has often been defined as a manifestation of extramural spread particularly on CT criteria (Thoeni *et al.* 1981; van Waes *et al.* 1983). In our experience, this was nearly always a manifestation of desmoplastic response and represented fibrosis rather than tumour extension. Of note was the fact that this desmoplastic response occurred maximally where the tumour had formed an ulcer and not at the level of the invading tumour mass. This may relate to the observation that desmoplasia does not occur at the invasive margin and may represent the host response to tumour limiting its extension when this is present (Hewitt *et al.* 1993). Its distinct appearance on MRI as being of much lower signal and forming fine strands into perirectal fat is valuable in distinguishing this from tumour. Peritumoral fibrosis has a distinct MR appearance that can be distinguished from the tumour itself. Fibrosis has a lower signal and is spiculated, as opposed to the broad-based pushing or nodular configuration of an advancing tumour margin. A potential source of overstaging is the confusion between tumour and inflammation. An inflammatory reaction at the growing tumour margin, following the contour of the tumour itself, occurs in about 25 per cent of rectal cancers (Jass 1986), but this is usually of the order of microns, rather than millimetres, in thickness (Svennevig *et al.* 1984), and insufficient to result in significant overstaging. MR has the potential to overstage or understage borderline T3/T2 tumours, as noted by others using an endorectal coil (Schnall & Kressel 1994). However, it is arguable as to whether differentiating between minimal T3 infiltration and T2 lesions is of consequence in patient management as it is known that patients with minimal T3 infiltration into perirectal fat are of low risk of surgical failure from circumferential excision margin involvement. The main advantage of thin-slice MRI is its accurate assessment of extramural spread that reflects the extent of spread on subsequent histology. The reliable pre-operative assessment of tumour depth should help to identify T3 patients in whom adjuvant therapy would not offer an advantage, such as those with minimally invasive T3 tumours and T2 lesions.

Assessment of pathological prognostic factors

Thin slice MRI staging is not just limited to an assessment of the TNM status. Careful correlation of histopathology wholemount section with specimen MR and pre-operative MR images demonstrated that other pathological prognostic factors could be identified pre-operatively (Brown *et al.* 1998). Tumour nodules are identified if deposits of either identical signal intensity as the primary tumour or mixed signal intensity are shown in the mesorectal fat (Figure 7.2). In this author's experience, size is not useful as a criterion for lymph node involvement since this will result in overstaging in patients with benign nodal reactive hyperplasia; however, a lymph node is classified as normal if it has smooth sharply demarcated borders and returns high signal. Extramural vascular invasion can be identified as serpiginous tumour extension into perirectal fat and along the perirectal vessels (Figure 7.3). The distance of tumour to the anal sphincter may be measured by locating the lowermost slice containing tumour on the sagittal T2 weighted images and measuring the distance to the upper edge of the anal sphincter complex. Thin-slice MRI can demonstrate the relationship of tumour to the peritoneal reflection, as well as the presence of tumour penetration through the serosa at or above the peritoneal reflection.

Thin-slice MRI correctly identifies both tumours with anal sphincter invasion and patients with distal tumour extension to within 1.5 cm of the edge of the sphincter (Brown *et al.* 1998). MRI also correctly predicts the relationship of the tumour to the peritoneal reflection and correctly identifies all tumours lying at or above the peritoneal reflection. Peritoneal infiltration is characterised by the identification of nodular extension of tumour through the peritoneal reflection. The depiction of irregular foci of tumour signal within the mesorectum correlates with tumour

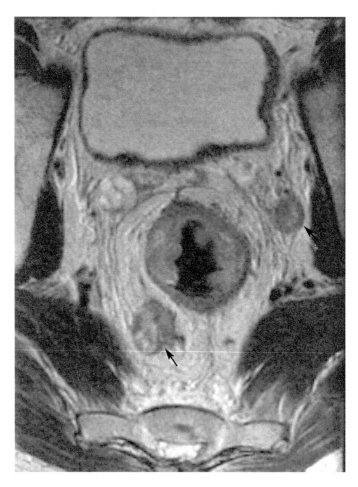

Figure 7.2 Axial T2 weighted high-resolution image demonstrating extramural tumour deposits (arrows). Tumour deposits are recognised by their mixed signal intensity and irregular borders

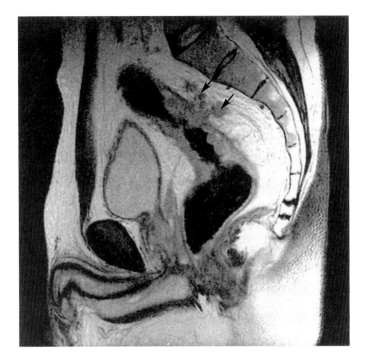

Figure 7.3 Sagittal T2 weighted scan through rectum, showing extramural extension of tumour along the superior rectal vessels (arrow). This correlated with extramural venous invasion

mesorectal deposits or lymph node involvement. The main limitation of any of the current staging modalities is the inability to detect microscopic or partial nodal involvement, although Oberg *et al.* (1998) have shown that micrometastases are not a useful prognostic marker. Future developments in MRI such as lymph node-specific contrast agents may improve the detection of this small subset of patients with lymph node involvement without significant extramural spread.

Conclusions

The potential value of thin-slice, high-resolution MRI of the pelvis is in assessing the important surgical prognostic risk factors. In the local staging of rectal cancer high resolution MRI should be used not only to predict the T stage but also to assess: the depth of extramural spread of tumour, the relationship of tumour to the peritoneal reflection and to the anal sphincter complex, the relationship between the outermost extension of tumour and the mesorectal fascia, the presence and location of mesorectal deposits, and to identify other prognostic factors, such as extramural venous invasion and peritoneal invasion. Pre-operative identification of patients with adverse prognostic features may allow targeting of such patients for the most appropriate pre-operative adjuvant therapy, assist in surgical planning and serve as an accurate baseline study from which to assess the success of different treatment strategies.

Acknowledgements

The Rectal Cancer High Resolution MRI Project was funded by grants from BUPA in association with the Royal College of Radiologists and Wales NHS Research and Development.

The author would like to thank the following collaborators for their input into this project: Dr J Blethyn, Dr MW Bourne, Dr NS Dallimore, Dr TS Maughan, Dr RG Newcombe, Dr C Phillips, Mr AG Radcliffe, Dr CJ Richards and Dr GT Williams.

References

Adam IJ, Mohamdee MO, Martin IG, Scott N, Finan PJ, Johnston D, Dixon MF & Quirke P (1994). Role of circumferential margin involvement in the local recurrence of rectal cancer. *Lancet* **344**, 707–11.

Adams DR, Blatchford GJ, Lin KM, Ternent CA, Thorsen AG, Christensen MA (1999). Use of preoperative ultrasound staging for treatment of rectal cancer. *Diseases of the Colon and Rectum* **42**, 159-66.

Akasu T, Sugihara K, Moriya Y & Fujita S (1997). Limitations and pitfalls of transrectal ultrasonography for staging of rectal cancer. *Diseases of the Colon & Rectum* **40**, S10–S15.

Baigrie RJ & Berry AR (1994). Management of advanced rectal cancer. *British Journal of Surgery* **81**, 343–52.

Beynon J (1994). Rectum in ultrasound in gastroenterology. *Clinics in Diagnostic Ultrasound* vol.29 (ed. PA Dubbins & AEA Joseph), p.169. Churchill Livingstone, Edinburgh.

Brown G, Richards CJ, Radcliffe AG, PD Carey, Bourne MW & Williams GT (1996). High resolution MRI: a promising technique for preoperative staging in rectal cancer. *Gut* **39**(suppl.1), 44.

Brown G, Richards CJ, Radcliffe AG, Carey PD, Bourne MW & Williams GT (1998). MRI of surgical prognostic factors in rectal cancer. *Radiology* **209**, 252.

Brown G, Richards C, Dallimore NS, Radcliffe AG, Carey PD, Bourne MW & Williams GT (1999). Rectal carcinoma: thin section MR imaging for staging in 28 patients. *Radiology* **211**, 215–22.

Cawthorn SJ, Parums DV, Gibbs NM, A'Hern RP, Caffarey SM, Broughton CI *et al.* (1990). Extent of mesorectal spread and involvement of lateral resection margin as prognostic factors after surgery for rectal cancer. *Lancet* **335**, 1055–9.

Cedermark B, Johansson H, Reiger A, Rutqvist LE, Theve T & Wilking N (1990). Preoperative short-term radiotherapy in operable rectal carcinoma. a prospective randomised trial. *Cancer* **66**, 49–55.

Cedermark B , Johansson H, Reiger A, Rutqvist LE, Theve T & Wilking N (1994). The Stockholm II trial on preoperative short term radiotherapy in operable rectal carcinoma – a prospective randomised trial. *Proceedings of the American Society of Clinical Oncology*, 198

Cedermark B, Johansson H, Rutqvist LE & Wilking N (1995). The Stockholm I trial of preoperative short term radiotherapy in operable rectal carcinoma. A prospective randomized trial. Stockholm Colorectal Cancer Study Group. *Cancer* **75**, 2269–75.

Chung CK, Stryker JA & Demuth WE (1983). Patterns of failure following surgery alone for colorectal carcinoma. *Journal of Surgical Oncology* **22**, 65–70.

Dahlberg M, Glimelius B, Graf W & Pahlman L (1998). Preoperative irradiation affects functional results after surgery for rectal cancer: results from a randomized study. *Diseases of the Colon & Rectum* **41**, 543–9; discussion 549–51.

Dukes CE (1932). The classification of cancer of the rectum. *Journal of Pathology* **35**, 323–32.

Durdey P & Williams NS (1992). Pre-operative evaluation of patients with low rectal carcinoma [Review] [65 refs]. *World Journal of Surgery* **16**, 430–6.

Frykholm GJ, Pahlman L & Glimelius B (1995). Treatment of local recurrences of rectal carcinoma. *Radiotherapy and Oncology* **34**, 185–94.

Gerard A, Buyse M, Nordlinger B *et al.* (1988). Preoperative radiotherapy as adjuvant treatment in rectal cancer. final results of a randomised study of The European Organisation for Research and Treatment of Cancer (EORTC). *Annals of Surgery* **208**, 606–14.

Harrison JC, Dean PJ, el-Zeky F & Vander Zwaag R (1994). From Dukes through Jass: pathological prognostic indicators in rectal cancer. *Human Pathology* **25**, 498–505.

Heald RJ, Husband EM & Ryall RD (1982). The mesorectum in rectal cancer surgery – the clue to pelvic recurrence? *British Journal of Surgery* **69**, 613–16.

Heald RJ & Ryall RD (1986). Recurrence and survival after total mesorectal excision for rectal cancer. *Lancet* **1**, 1479–82.

Heald RJ, Moran BJ, Ryall RD, Sexton R & MacFarlane JK (1998). Rectal cancer: the Basingstoke experience of total mesorectal excision, 1978–1997. *Archives of Surgery* **133**, 894–9.

Hewitt RE, Powe DG & Carter IG *et al.* (1993). Desmoplasia and relevance to colorectal tumour invasion. *International Journal of Cancer* **53**, 62–9.

Hida J, Yasutomi M, Maruyama T, Fujimoto K, Uchida T & Okuno K (1997). Lymph node metastases detected in the mesorectum distal to carcinoma of the rectum by the clearing method: justification of total mesorectal excision. *Journal of the American College of Surgeons* **184**, 584–8.

Janjan NA, Khoo VS, Abbruzzese J, Pazdur R, Dubrow R, Cleary KR, Allen PK, Lynch PM, Glober G, Wolff R, Rich TA & Skibber J (1999). Tumor downstaging and sphincter preservation with preoperative chemoradiation in locally advanced rectal cancer: the MD Anderson Cancer Center experience. *International Journal of Radiation Oncology, Biology, Physics* **44**, 1027–38.

Jass JR (1986). Lymphocytic infiltration and survival in rectal cancer. *Journal of Clinical Pathology* **39**, 585–9.

Jass JR (1995). Prognostic factors in rectal cancer. *European Journal of Cancer* **31**A, 862–3.

Jass JR, Atkin WS, Cuzick J, Bussey HJ, Morson BC, Northover JM *et al.* (1986). The grading of rectal cancer: historical perspectives and a multivariate analysis of 447 cases. *Histopathology* **10**, 437–59.

Jass JR, Love SB & Northover JM (1987). A new prognostic classification of rectal cancer. *Lancet* **1**, 1303–6.

Kim NK, Kim MJ, Yun SH, Sohn SK & Min JS (1999). Comparative study of transrectal ultrasonography, pelvic computerized tomography, and magnetic resonance imaging in preoperative staging of rectal cancer. *Diseases of the Colon & Rectum* **42**, 770–5.

Kusunoki M, Yanagi H, Kamikonya N, Hishikawa Y, Shoji Y & Yamamura T (1994). Preoperative detection of local extension of carcinoma of the rectum using magnetic resonance imaging. *Journal of The American College of Surgeons* **179**, 653–6.

Lindmark G, Elvin A, Pahlman L & Glimelius B (1992). The value of preoperative endosonography in preoperative staging of rectal cancer. *International Journal of Colorectal Disease* **7**, 162–6

Lindmark G, Gerdin B, Pahlman L, Bergstrom R & Glimelius B (1994). Prognostic predictors in colorectal cancer. *Diseases of the Colon & Rectum* **37**, 1219–27.

Macnicholas MMJ, Joyce WP, Dolan J, Gibney RG, Macerlaine DP & Hyland J (1994). Magnetic resonance imaging of rectal carcinoma: a prospective study. *British Journal of Surgery* **81**, 911–14.

Maier AG, Barton PP, Neuhold NR, Herbst F, Teleky BK & Lechner GL (1997). Peritumoral tissue reaction at transrectal US as a possible cause of overstaging in rectal cancer: histopathologic correlation. *Radiology* **203**, 785–9.

Maldjian C, Smith R, Kilger A, Schnall M, Ginsberg G, Kochman M (2000). Endorectal surface coil MR imaging as a staging technique for rectal carcinoma: a comparison study to rectal endosonography. *Abdominal Imaging* **25**, 75–80.

Marsh PJ, James RD & Schofield PF (1994). Adjuvant preoperative radiotherapy for locally advanced rectal carcinoma. Results of a prospective, randomized trial. *Diseases of Colon & Rectum* **37**, 1205–14.

Massari M, De Simone M, Cioffi U, Rosso L, Chiarelli M, Gabrielli F (1998). Value and limits of endorectal ultrasonography for preoperative staging of rectal carcinoma. *Surgical Laparoscopy, Endoscopy and Percutaneous Techniques* **8**, 438–44.

Mehta S, Johnson RJ & Schofield PF (1994). Staging of colorectal cancer [Review]. *Clinical Radiology* **49**, 515–23.

Minsky BD, Cohen AM, Enker WE, Saltz L, Guillem JG, Paty PB, Kelsen DP, Kemeny N, Ilson D, Bass J & Conti J (1997). Preoperative 5-FU, low-dose leucovorin, and radiation therapy for locally advanced and unresectable rectal cancer. *International Journal of Radiation Oncology, Biology, Physics* **37**, 289–95.

Oberg A, Stenling R, Tavelin B & Lindmark G (1998). Are lymph node micrometastases of any clinical significance in Dukes Stages A and B colorectal cancer? *Diseases of the Colon & Rectum* **41**, 1244–9.

Pahlman L & Glimelius B (1995). The value of adjuvant radio(chemo)therapy for rectal cancer. *European Journal of Cancer* **31**A, 1347–50.

Schnall MD & Kressel HY (1994). Rectal tumour stage: correlation of endorectal MR imaging and pathologic findings. *Radiology* **190**, 709–14.

Shepherd NA, Baxter KJ & Love SB (1995). Influence of local peritoneal involvement on pelvic recurrence and prognosis in rectal cancer [see comments]. *Journal of Clinical Pathology* **48**, 849–55.

Svennevig JL, Lunde OC, Holter J & Bjørgsvik D (1984). Lymphoid infiltration and prognosis in colorectal carcinoma. *British Journal of Cancer* **49**, 375–7.

Talbot IC, Ritchie S, Leighton M, Hughes AO, Bussey HJ & Morson BC (1981). Invasion of veins by carcinoma of rectum: method of detection, histological features and significance. *Histopathology* **5**, 141–63.

Thaler W, Watzka S, Martin F, La Guardia G, Psenner K, Bonatti *et al.* (1994). Preoperative staging of rectal cancer by endoluminal ultrasound vs magnetic resonance imaging. *Diseases of the Colon & Rectum* 37, 1189–93.

Thoeni RF, Moss AA, Schnyder P *et al.* (1981). Detection and staging of primary rectal and rectosigmoid cancer by computed tomography. *Radiology* **141**, 135–8.

Ueno H, Mochizuki H & Tamakuma S (1998). Prognostic significance of extranodal microscopic foci discontinuous with primary lesion in rectal cancer. *Diseases of the Colon & Rectum* **41**, 55–61.

van Waes PF, Koehler PR & Feldberg MA (1983). Management of rectal carcinoma: impact of computed tomography. *American Journal of Roentgenology* **140**, 1137–42.

Vauthey JN, Marsh RW, Zlotecki RA, Abdalla EK, Solorzano CC, Bray EJ, Freeman ME, Lauwers GY, Kubilis PS, Mendenhall WM & Copeland EM 3rd (1999). Recent advances in the treatment and outcome of locally advanced rectal cancer. *Annals of Surgery* **229**, 745–52.

Verschueren RC, Mulder NH, Hooykaas JA, Szabo BG & Karrenbeld A (1998). Pelvic exenteration for advanced primary rectal cancer in male patients. *Clinical Oncology (Royal College of Radiologists)* **10**, 318–21.

Wheeler JM, Warren BF, Jones AC, Mortensen NJ (1999). Preoperative radiotherapy for rectal cancer: implications for surgeons, pathologists and radiologists. *British Journal of Surgery* **86**, 1108–20.

Yasutomi M (1997). Advances in rectal cancer surgery in Japan. *Diseases of the Colon & Rectum* **40**(suppl.), S74–9.

Zerhouni EA, Rutter C, Hamilton SR *et al.* (1996). CT and MR imaging in the staging of colorectal carcinoma: report of the Radiology Diagnostic Oncology Group II. *Radiology* **200**, 443–51.

Chapter 8

Could chemoradiation make the surgeon redundant in rectal cancer?

David Sebag-Montefiore

Introduction

In the past decade, randomised controlled trials have demonstrated improved outcome for concurrent chemoradiotherapy (CRT) when compared with radiotherapy alone as definitive treatment of anal (Anonymous 1996a; Bartelink *et al.* 1997), oesophageal (al-Sarraf *et al.* 1997) and cervical cancer (Morris *et al.* 1999). In addition, there is also evidence of improved survival with the use of pre-operative CRT in cervical and oesophageal cancer (Walsh *et al.* 1996; Keys *et al.* 1999).

The development of an optimal concurrent CRT regimen should be through careful phase I/II studies in patients with assessable disease prior to testing in the pre-operative setting. The promotion of a pre-operative combined-modality approach to definitive treatment is best illustrated by the stepwise development of concurrent CRT in squamous cell carcinoma of the anus. The possible application of this approach to rectal cancer will then be discussed.

The anal cancer story

Although the management of squamous cell carcinoma of the anal canal in the UK consisted of radical abdomino-perineal excision of the anorectum (APER) until well into the 1980s, enthusiastic and dedicated radiotherapists such as Jean Papillon demonstrated the ability of radiotherapy to produce durable local control (Papillon *et al.* 1983). The radiotherapy techniques combined external beam radiotherapy and brachytherapy with a fine balance between tumour control and late normal tissue morbidity with the need for specific skills in brachytherapy techniques. Thus although radiotherapy alone was accepted by a minority of clinicians as acceptable definitive treatment, radical surgery remained the accepted standard.

The first step

The first step in the development of concurrent CRT was the pioneering work of a North American surgeon, Norman Nigro. Nigro published a preliminary report in 1974 (Nigro *et al.* 1993) of three patients treated with a regimen of external beam radiotherapy (EBRT) of 30.0–34.7 Gy over three to five weeks with proferimycin (1 patient), and mitomycin C (2 patients) given on the first day of radiotherapy and a five-day infusion of 5-fluorouracil (5-FU) given during the first week of radiotherapy.

An abdominoperineal resection was planned for six weeks after completion of radiotherapy. Complete clinical response was documented in all three patients six to eight weeks after completion of radiotherapy. Two patients underwent APER with histological evidence of pathological complete response (pCR) and one patient refused APER. All three patients were disease-free with a follow-up of 6, 13, and 14 months respectively.

Nigro's group subsequently published (Leichman *et al.* 1985) a larger cohort of 45 patients treated with 30 Gy EBRT, a single-dose mitomycin on day 1 and 1 g/m²/d by continuous infusion of 5-FU on days 1–4 and 29–32. APER was planned for six weeks later. Importantly, five of the first six patients achieved pCR and the surgery was significantly modified to full thickness biopsy, restricting APER to those patients with viable residual malignancy on biopsy. Thirty-eight (84%) patients were found to have no evidence of malignancy on biopsy and with a median follow-up of 50 months, 34 (89%) patients remained disease-free. This publication demonstrated a very high complete clinical response rate to CRT, allowing APER to be reserved as salvage therapy for patients with evidence of residual malignancy on the basis of post-treatment biopsy.

Confirmatory studies

Further evidence of the dramatic results reported by Nigro were then required. A number of workers provided this evidence. In particular, Cummings *et al.* (1991) in Toronto reported their experience of 192 patients treated between 1958 and 1989 in a total of seven sequential studies using different radiotherapy fractionation, continuous and split-course treatments and concurrent chemotherapy schedules using 5-FU either alone or in combination with Mitomycin. Although the numbers of patients in individual protocols were small, it appeared that the combination of mitomycin C, 5-FU and EBRT resulted in the highest rates of local control.

It has been a major success of non-surgical oncological research that three successful randomised controlled trials of a combined total of 1,005 patients were successfully completed in a disease as rare as anal cancer between 1987 and 1994. The United Kindgom Coordinating Committee for Cancer Research (UKCCCR) trial (Anonymous 1996a) and the European Organization for Research and Treatment of Cancer (EORTC) radiotherapy trial (Bartelink *et al.* 1997) established that CRT using mitomycin C and 5-FU was superior to radiotherapy alone for the end points of local control and colostomy-free survival. The Radiation Therapy and Oncology Group (RTOG) and Eastern Cooperative Oncology Group (ECOG) trial (Flam *et al.* 1996) demonstrated that CRT using mitomycin C and 5-FU was superior to 5-FU for the end point of colostomy-free survival.

It is of critical importance that the earlier phase I and phase II studies, which demonstrated high complete clinical response following CRT, allowed the initial planned approach of APER in phase I and phase II studies to be rapidly relegated to the role of salvage surgery. The successful launch and subsequent results from the phase III randomised trials effectively signalled the retreat of the surgeon (Northover 1991) in the primary management of squamous cell carcinoma of the anal canal.

Chemoradiotherapy in rectal cancer

Paradoxically the development of CRT in rectal cancer has until recently taken place in the post-operative setting. Two randomised controlled trials following potentially curative resection of rectal cancer have demonstrated improved local control (Krook *et al.* 1991) and survival (Krook *et al.* 1991; O'Connell *et al.* 1994). However, in the majority of patients who are considered to have resectable rectal cancer, there is considerable uncertainty surrounding the optimal adjuvant radiotherapy policy (Steele & Sebag-Montefiore 2000).

Pre-operative radiotherapy in locally advanced disease

Patients with locally advanced rectal cancer provide a subgroup in which pre-operative radiotherapy and CRT can be refined in phase I, II and, ultimately, phase III trials. The interpretation of phase II results is confounded by the wide heterogeneity of local disease extent, the lack of radiological response assessment and variation in the quality of surgery. Almost all studies consist of a combined-modality approach of pre-operative radiotherapy or CRT followed by radical surgery.

There are considerable difficulties in the local staging of rectal cancer. Transrectal ultrasound (TRUS) is useful in assessing the stage of the primary tumour in resectable disease and is most useful in identifying the small subgroup of patients suitable for local excision. In locally advanced disease, MRI is useful in anatomically demonstrating the extent of disease for the purposes of radiotherapy target volume definition. However, both techniques are unable accurately to predict microscopic lymph node involvement.

A major problem in interpreting the published literature of pre-operative radiotherapy studies is the lack of any agreed classification of local disease extent. For example, the assessment of tumour mobility does not describe the volume of tumour. Even the description of a fixed inoperable tumour applies to a widely heterogeneous local extent of disease, ranging from a small tumour fixed, for example, anteriorly locally invading the prostate, to a massive tumour filling the true pelvis and confirmed to be fixed in all planes and confirmed to be inoperable at laparotomy.

An assessment of the impact of pre-operative non-surgical treatment can be made by comparing the pre-treatment assessment with the histopathological stage of the resected specimen. This is commonly reported in the published literature as the proportion of resections with histopathological complete response (pCR) and T1,2 N0 disease. This information must, however, be interpreted with caution according to the local extent of disease. To illustrate this point, a 20 per cent pCR rate is impressive if the study group consists of fixed, inoperable tumours. A similar pCR rate is less impressive if the study group consists of small, mobile tumours where a proportion of patients may have T1–2 N0 tumours prior to treatment.

Downstaging using pre-operative radiotherapy alone

The published literature for the use of pre-operative radiotherapy alone demonstrates a fairly wide range in total radiation dose of 30–60 Gy with many reports reflecting changes in dose and fractionation during the period studied (Tobin *et al.* 1991; Kerman *et al.* 1992; Mendenhall *et al.* 1992; Ahmad & Nagle 1997; Berger *et al.* 1997; Lusinchi *et al.* 1997; Kaminsky-Forrett *et al.* 1998; Mohiuddin *et al.* 1998; Wagman *et al.* 1998). There is also heterogeneity in the local extent of disease, although the majority of reports include a proportion of patients with resectable or mobile disease with the intention of increasing the chance of sphincter-preserving surgery. It is disappointing therefore that the reported pCR rate in the resected specimen ranges from 3 to 11 per cent (Tobin *et al.* 1991; Kerman *et al.* 1992; Mendenhall *et al.* 1992; Ahmad & Nagle 1997; Berger *et al.* 1997; Lusinchi *et al.* 1997; Kaminsky-Forrett *et al.* 1998; Mohiuddin *et al.* 1998; Wagman *et al.* 1998).

Further information is available from randomised controlled trials. The MRC CR02 trial (Anonymous 1996b) randomised 279 patients with partially or completely fixed rectal cancer between initial surgery and pre-operative radiotherapy using a total dose of 40 Gy. Although no information is presented on whether pCR was seen, 16 per cent of patients who received pre-operative radiotherapy had Dukes' A tumours compared with 7 per cent who underwent initial surgery. Two similar randomised trials in resectable rectal cancer found pCR rates of 4.5 per cent (Dahl *et al.* 1990) and 3 per cent (Gerard *et al.* 1988), using total doses of 31.5–34.5 Gy of pre-operative radiotherapy.

Pre-operative CRT

With such low rates of pCR with radiotherapy alone and following the success of CRT in squamous cell carcinoma of the anus, it is logical to evaluate the role of pre-operative CRT in rectal cancer. The majority of studies incorporated 5-FU (with or without folinic acid) with radiotherapy and studied patients with locally advanced, fixed or recurrent disease.

There have been very few phase I studies prospectively evaluating either the optimal 5-FU dose in combination with a fixed total dose of radiotherapy or, alternatively, a dose escalation study of radiotherapy dose against a fixed dose of chemotherapy. Minsky *et al.* (1992) have reported two parallel phase I studies using high-dose folinic acid, 50.4 Gy of irradiation and two dose levels of 5-FU (200 mg/m^2 and 250 mg/m^2). One study group consisted of patients with unresectable disease who received pre-operative CRT and the second group consisted of patients receiving post-operative radiotherapy.

Bosset *et al.* (1993) performed three sequential phase II studies using a fixed dose of 45 Gy in 25 fractions with de-escalation of 5-FU/FA given on days 1–5 and 29–33. A total of 85 patients were treated, of whom 37 were primarily unresectable, 13 locally recurrent, 15 patients had gross residual disease after surgery and 20 had potentially resectable disease. Regression curve analysis, using either grade 3 or greater toxicity or incomplete treatment as an end point against the 5-FU dose, determined the 5-FU dose for use in a phase III trial as 350 mg/m^2. It is important to note that 5-FU was given as a short infusion prior to radiotherapy. A pCR rate of 14 per cent was found in the 43 patients who underwent resection.

Rich *et al.* (1995) using infusional 5-FU 300 mg/m^2/day given five days per week with 45 Gy in 25 fractions of pelvic radiotherapy, treated 77 patients with operable T3 rectal cancer with pre-operative CRT. Histopathological staging included a pCR rate of 29 per cent with a further 35 per cent of patients with T1–2 N0 disease. Local failure was seen in only three of 77 patients after a median follow-up of 27 months. The recently published analysis of outcome in this relatively homogeneous group of patients with resectable rectal cancer, of whom 92 per cent had T3 disease, demonstrates significantly improved outcome for patients with pCR as well as those with T1,2 N0 disease and a poor outcome for the minority of patients who fail to respond to CRT (Janjan *et al.* 1999).

Further studies are required that assess the impact of pre-operative CRT in the resected specimen. Mandard and colleagues published a scoring system to assess the impact of pre-operative radiotherapy on the resected oesophageal resection specimen (Mandard *et al.* 1994). The use of this or similar grading systems is required in assessing rectal cancer specimens. Alternative approaches would include the assessment of apoptotis (Scott *et al.* 1998) or studies that assay the expression of thymidylate synthase, thymidine phosphorylase and topoisomerase in the biopsy specimen and whether they can predict the impact of pre-operative CRT.

Acute toxicity of CRT using 5-FU

The need for future phase I/II studies integrating the synchronous delivery of combination chemotherapy with radiotherapy is illustrated by examples of high levels of acute toxicity reported in some studies using 5-FU that may also prevent delivery of the full planned dose of radiotherapy.

Cooper *et al.* (1993) using a weekly 5-FU FA bolus regimen reported 38 per cent grade 3–4 toxicity, and 26 per cent of patient did not receive the planned radiotherapy total dose of 45 Gy. Glynne-Jones (personal communication) found that a short infusion of 350 mg/m^2 of 5-FU with low-dose FA given on days 1–5 and 29–33 combined with 45 Gy radiotherapy resulted in grade 3–4 toxicity in 1/14 (7 per cent) patients, whereas 5/6 (83 per cent) experienced such toxicity when the same dose of 5-FU was given as a bolus.

Rich *et al.* (1995) demonstrated that 300 mg/m^2/day of infusional 5-FU could be given five days per week during pre-operative radiotherapy, whereas a lower dose of infusional 5-FU would be required if the 5-FU was given continuously.

However, low-grade 3–4 acute toxicity (less than 10 per cent) and high levels of radiotherapy compliance (full dose of planned radiotherapy received in over 95 per cent of patients) may be achieved using validated short- or continuous-infusion 5-FU with a total dose of 45 Gy of planned radiotherapy (Sebag-Montefiore & Glynne-Jones 1997).

Outcome following pre-operative CRT using 5-FU

Most published reports of pre-operative CRT provide data on acute toxicity and histopathological stage but commonly lack mature outcome data. Bosset *et al.* (2000) have recently reported mature outcome data of 66 patients with resectable rectal cancer defined as either stage uT3 on transrectal ultrasound, circumferential or tethered treated with pre-op CRT. Sixty patients underwent resection, of whom 9 (15 per cent) had pT0 and 17 (28 per cent) had pTis-pT2 N0 disease. After a mean follow-up of 4.5 years, the five-year pelvic disease-free survival was 92 per cent in the whole group, including the patients who did not undergo resection. The authors comment that the high rate of pelvic control was obtained without specifying surgical technique, and state that total mesorectal excision (TME) 'was not performed.'

There are relatively few phase III trials evaluating the role of pre-op CRT. The EORTC 22921 trial is randomising patients with resectable T3 and T4 non-metastatic rectal cancer between pre-operative radiotherapy and pre-operative CRT with a second randomisation between post-operative adjuvant chemotherapy and no chemotherapy.

In the USA the NSABP R03 trial which has closed owing to poor recruitment, randomised patients between a pre-operative and post-operative regimen consisting of sequential and concurrent chemotherapy with radiotherapy. A preliminary report (Hyams *et al.* 1997) of the first 116 patients recruited in this trial reported a pCR using the pre-operative approach of 8 per cent and a higher rate of sphincter preservation. In the pre-operative CRT arm 47 per cent of patients underwent anterior resection compared with 28 per cent in the initial surgery arm.

Conclusions of CRT using 5-FU

At present the low rate of pCR restricts CRT to a pre-operative approach followed by radical surgery. The EORTC trial will help to determine the future control arm for subsequent pre-operative CRT phase III trials in rectal cancer.

Future combination CRT regimens

The improvements in response rates and progression-free survival demonstrated in studies of combination chemotherapy compared with 5-FU regimens in metastatic disease are summarised in Chapter 5 of this volume. This suggests that the careful integration of a second chemotherapy drug may result in improved clinical and histopathological complete response rates.

There is limited experience of the addition of cisplatin to 5-FU using pre-operative CRT. Chari *et al.* (1995) used 5-FU 500 mg/m^2 as a rapid infusion followed by cisplatin 20 mg/m^2 days 1–5 and 29–33 combined with 45 Gy of EBRT given pre-operatively in 43 patients with resectable disease. Twenty-two patients were considered to have complete response on sigmoidoscopy, although following resection 11 (27 per cent) specimens were free of tumour (pCR). There was, however, significant associated toxicity with this regimen. Six patients were described to have haematological toxicity. Of greater concern was diarrhoea requiring protocol alteration, with grade 4 diarrhoea, occurring in three (7 per cent) patients, requiring interruption of the protocol for two or more weeks and a further 5 (12 per cent) patients with moderate diarrhoea, who required a 20 per cent reduction in the 5-FU dose. Post-operative morbidity included prolonged perineal drainage in 49 per cent of patients and a further 10 per cent with perineal dehiscence. The toxicity of this CRT regimen is of concern. The use of an uncommon 5-FU CRT regimen whose baseline toxicity is not well documented with the addition of a second chemotherapy drug may account for the toxicity seen and emphasises the need for the stepwise development of the combination CRT schedules.

In contrast, building on their previous experience of the use of a four-day continuous infusion given during the first and fifth week of EBRT, Valentini *et al.* (1999a) added cisplatin 60 mg/m^2 on days 1 and 29 in 40 patients described to have resectable disease, although tethering was present in 82 per cent of them. This regimen was associated with a 5 per cent acute grade 3–4 toxicity. The histopathological outcome demonstrated pCR in nine (23 per cent), pT1–2 in 15 (37 per cent) and Tmic in four (10 per cent) patients where Tmic was defined as rare isolated residual cancer cells. An increase by more than 2 cm of the distance between the anorectal ring and the inferior extent of tumour was found in 9 (23 per cent) of the patients. This important information illustrates how the use of pre-op CRT may increase the rate of sphincter-preserving resections performed, although mature outcome data are still required to determine whether this is associated with an acceptably low incidence of local recurrence.

A number of trial groups are currently performing phase I studies combining the newer chemotherapy drugs in combination with pre-operative radiotherapy. It is essential that there is meticulous attention to both chemotherapy and radiotherapy quality assurance and adherence to protocol.

Early reports were presented in abstract form at the American Society of Clinical Oncology (ASCO) meeting in May 1999. Early reports of phase I studies include the combination of EBRT pre-operatively with UFT (Feliu *et al.* 1999; Hoff *et al.* 1999), raltitrexed (James *et al.* 1999; Valentini *et al.* 1999b), irinotecan (Minsky *et al.* 1999) and irinotecan combined with continuous-infusion 5-FU (Mitchell *et al.* 1999). The Colorectal Clinical Oncology Group (CCOG) (Glynne-Jones *et al.* 2000) and other trial groups are also performing phase I studies evaluating the addition of oxaliplatin to 5-FU and EBRT.

Conclusions

The use of pre-operative CRT using 5-FU regimens is only suitable as a pre-operative approach prior to surgical resection. The encouraging results of combination chemotherapy in metastatic disease can only be translated into safe CRT regimens through carefully conducted phase I and phase II trials. Only when phase II studies have demonstrated acceptable acute toxicity and some early evidence of improved response will phase III trials make it possible to test these novel regimens.

There is an opportunity to evaluate the use of validated combination CRT regimens in patients who require abdomino-perineal excision as pre-operative treatment prior to resection. It is far too early to predict whether such combination CRT regimens will produce the dramatic and durable complete responses that have been achieved in anal cancer.

For the next few years at least pre-operative CRT does not pose a major threat to the role of the surgeon in resecting rectal cancer. The benefits in terms of sphincter preservation, functional outcome, local control and survival are likely to come from further trials that evaluate the multidisciplinary management integrating resection with adjuvant radiotherapy and chemotherapy.

References

Ahmad NR & Nagle D (1997). Long-term results of preoperative radiation therapy alone for stage T3 and T4 rectal cancer. *British Journal of Surgery* **84**, 1445–8.

al-Sarraf M, Martz K, Herskovic A, Leichman L, Brindle JS, Vaitkevicius VK, Cooper J, Byhardt R, Davis L & Emami B (1997). Progress report of combined chemoradiotherapy versus radiotherapy alone in patients with esophageal cancer: an intergroup study. *Journal of Clinical Oncology* **15**, 277–84.

Anonymous (1996a). Epidermoid anal cancer: results from the UKCCCR randomised trial of radiotherapy alone versus radiotherapy, 5-fluorouracil, and mitomycin. UKCCCR Anal Cancer Trial Working Party. UK Co-ordinating Committee on Cancer *Lancet* **348**, 1049–54.

Anonymous (1996b). Randomised trial of surgery alone versus radiotherapy followed by surgery for potentially operable locally advanced rectal cancer. Medical Research Council Rectal Cancer Working Party. *Lancet* **348**, 1605–10.

Bartelink H, Roelofsen F, Eschwege F, Rougier P, Bosset JF, Gonzalez DG, Peiffert D, van Glabbeke M & Pierart M (1997). Concomitant radiotherapy and chemotherapy is superior to radiotherapy alone in the treatment of locally advanced anal cancer: results of a phase III randomized trial of the European Organization for Research and Treatment of Cancer Radiotherapy and Gastrointestinal Cooperative Groups. *Journal of Clinical Oncology* **15**, 2040–9.

Berger C, de Muret A, Garaud P, Chapet S, Bourlier P, Reynaud B, Dorval E, de Calan L, Huten N, le Folch O & Calais G (1997). Preoperative radiotherapy (RT) for rectal cancer: predictive factors of tumor downstaging and residual tumor cell density (RTCD): prognostic implications. *International Journal of Radiation Oncology, Biology, Physics* **37**, 619–27.

Bosset, JF, Magnin V, Maingnon P, Mantion G, Pelissier EP, Mercier M, Chaillard G & Horiot J-C (2000). Preoperative radiochemotherapy in rectal cancer:long term results of a phase II trial. *International Journal of Radiation Oncology, Biology, Physics* **46**, 323–7.

Bosset JF, Pavy JJ, Hamers HP, Horiot JC, Fabri MC, Rougier P, Eschwege F & Schraub S (1993). Determination of the optimal dose of 5-fluorouracil when combined with low dose D,L-leucovorin and irradiation in rectal cancer: results of three consecutive phase II studies. EORTC Radiotherapy Group. *European Journal of Cancer* **29**A, 1406–10.

Chari RS, Tyler DS, Anscher MS, Russell L, Clary BM, Hathorn J & Seigler HF (1995). Preoperative radiation and chemotherapy in the treatment of adenocarcinoma of the rectum [see comments]. *Annals of Surgery* **221**, 778–86.

Cooper SG, Bonaventura A, Ackland SP, Joseph DJ, Stewart JF, Hamilton CS & Denham JW (1993). Pelvic radiotherapy with concurrent 5-fluorouracil modulated by leucovorin for rectal cancer: a phase II study. *Clinical Oncology (Royal College of Radiologists)* **5**, 169–73.

Cummings BJ, Keane TJ, O'Sullivan B, Wong CS & Catton CN (1991). Epidermoid anal cancer: treatment by radiation alone or by radiation and 5-fluorouracil with and without mitomycin C [see comments]. *International Journal of Radiation Oncology, Biology, Physics* **21**, 1115–25.

Dahl O, Horn A, Morild I, Halvorsen JF, Odland G, Reinertsen S, Reisaeter A, Kavli H & Thunold J (1990). Low-dose preoperative radiation postpones recurrences in operable rectal cancer. Results of a randomized multicenter trial in western Norway. [Review] [53 refs]. *Cancer* **66**, 2286–94.

Feliu J, Calvillo J, Escribano A, De Castro J, Espinosa E, Ordonez A, Zamora P, Garcia de Paredes ML, De las Heras B, Jiminez A & Gonzalez Baron M (1999). Neoadjuvant therapy of rectal carcinoma with UFT-folinic acid (LV) plus radiotherapy (RT). *Proceedings of the American Society of Clinical Oncology* **18**, 239a.

Flam M, John M, Pajak TF, Petrelli N, Myerson R, Doggett S, Quivey J, Rotman M, Kerman H, Coia L & Murray K (1996). Role of mitomycin in combination with fluorouracil and radiotherapy, and of salvage chemoradiation in the definitive nonsurgical treatment of epidermoid carcinoma of the anal canal: results of a phase III randomized intergroup study. *Journal of Clinical Oncology* **14**, 2527–39.

Gerard A, Buyse M, Nordlinger B, Loygue J, Pene F, Kempf P, Bosset JF, Gignoux M, Arnaud JP & Desaive C (1988). Preoperative radiotherapy as adjuvant treatment in rectal cancer. Final results of a randomized study of the European Organization for Research and Treatment of Cancer (EORTC). *Annals of Surgery* **208**, 606–14.

Glynne-Jones R, Falk S, Maughan T, Sebag-Montefiore D, Meadows HM, Das-Gupta A (2000). Results of pre-operative radiation and oxaliplatin in combination with 5 fluorouracil (5FU) and leucovorin (LV) in locally advanced rectal cancer: a pilot study. *Proceedings of the American Society of Clinical Oncology* **19**, 1225.

Hoff PM, Brito R, Slaughter M, Matei C, Lassere Y, Janjan N, Skibber J, Randolph J, Benner S & Pazdur R (1998). Preoperative UFT, oral leucovorin (LV) and radiotherapy (RT) for patients (pts) with resectable rectal carcinoma:an oral regimen with complete pathological responses. *Proceedings of the American Society of Clinical Oncology* **17**, 199.

Hyams DM, Mamounas EP, Petrelli N, Rockette H, Jones J, Wieand HS, Deutsch M, Wickerham L, Fisher B & Wolmark N (1997). A clinical trial to evaluate the worth of preoperative multimodality therapy in patients with operable carcinoma of the rectum: a progress report of National Surgical Breast and Bowel Project Protocol R-03. *Diseases of the Colon & Rectum* **40**, 131–9.

James RD, Price P & Smith M (1999). Raltitrexed ('Tomudex') plus radiotherapy is well tolerated and warrants further investigation in patients with advanced inoperable/recurrent rectal cancer. *Proceedings of the American Society of Clinical Oncology* **18**, 288a.

Janjan NA, Abbruzzese J, Pazdur R, Khoo VS, Cleary K, Dubrow R, Ajani J, Rich TA, Goswitz MS, Evetts PA, Allen PK, Lynch PM & Skibber JM (1999). Prognostic implications of response to preoperative infusional chemoradiation in locally advanced rectal cancer. *Radiotherapy & Oncology* **51**, 153–60.

Kaminsky-Forrett MC, Conroy T, Luporsi E, Peiffert D, Lapeyre M, Boissel Guillemin F & Bey P (1998). Prognostic implications of downstaging following preoperative radiation therapy for operable T3-T4 rectal cancer. *International Journal of Radiation Oncology, Biology, Physics* **42**, 935–41.

Kerman HD, Roberson SH, Bloom TS, Heron HC, Yaeger TE, Meese DL, Ritter AH, Tolland JT & Spangler AE (1992). Rectal carcinoma. Long-term experience with moderately high-dose preoperative radiation and low anterior resection. *Cancer* **69**, 2813–19.

Keys HM, Bundy BN, Stehman FB, Muderspach LI, Chafe WE, Suggs IIC, Walker JL, Gersell D & Mackey D (1999). Cisplatin, radiation, and adjuvant hysterectomy compared with radiation and adjuvant hysterectomy for bulky stage IB cervical carcinoma. *New England Journal of Medicine* **340**, 1154–61.

Krook JE, Moertel CG, Gunderson LL, Wieand HS, Collins RT, Beart RW, Kubista TP, Poon MA, Meyers WC & Mailliard JA (1991). Effective surgical adjuvant therapy for high-risk rectal carcinoma *New England Journal of Medicine* **324**, 709–15.

Leichman L, Nigro N, Vaitkevicius VK, Considine B, Buroker T, Bradley G, Seydel HG, Olchowski S, Cummings G & Leichman C (1985). Cancer of the anal canal. Model for preoperative adjuvant combined modality therapy. *American Journal of Medicine* **78**, 211–15.

Lusinchi A, Wibault P, Lasser P, Elias D, Bourrhis J, Rougier P, Ducreux M, Duvillard P & Eschwege F (1997). Abdominoperineal resection combined with pre- and postoperative radiation therapy in the treatment of low-lying rectal carcinoma. *International Journal of Radiation Oncology, Biology, Physics* **37**, 59–65.

Mandard AM, Dalibard F, Mandard JC, Marnay J, Henry-Amar M, Petiot JF, Roussel A, Jacob JH, Segol P & Samama (1994). Pathologic assessment of tumor regression after preoperative chemoradiotherapy of esophageal carcinoma. Clinicopathologic correlations. *Cancer* **73**, 2680–6.

Mendenhall WM, Bland KI, Copeland EM, Summers GE, Pfaff WW, Souba WW & Million RR (1992). Does preoperative radiation therapy enhance the probability of local control and survival in high-risk distal rectal cancer? *Annals of Surgery* **215**, 696–705.

Minsky BD, Cohen AM, Kemeny N, Enker WE, Kelsen DP, Reichman B, Saltz Sigurdson ER & Frankel J (1992). Combined modality therapy of rectal cancer: decreased acute toxicity with the preoperative approach. *Journal of Clinical Oncology* **10**, 1218–24.

Minsky BD, O'Reilly E, Wong D, Sharma S, Paty P, Guillem J, Cohen A, Ilson D, Hollywood E, Semple D, Kleban S, Kelsen D & Saltz LB (1999). Daily low-dose irinotecan (CPT-11) plus pelvic irradiation as preoperative treatment of locally advanced rectal cancer. *Proceedings of the American Society of Clinical Oncology* **18**, 266a.

Mitchell E, Ahmad N, Fry R, Anne PR, Rakinic J, Goldstein S, Rose L, Kaufman A, Hightower M, Palazzo J, Boman B, Bonanni R, Hoey D & Curran WJ (1999). Combined Modality Therapy of locally advanced or recurrent adenocarcinoma of the rectum: preliminary report of a phase I trial of chemotherapy (CT) with CPT-11, 5-FU and concomitant irradiation (RT). *Proceedings of the American Society of Clinical Oncology* **18**, 247a.

Mohiuddin M, Regine WF, Marks GJ & Marks JW (1998). High-dose preoperative radiation and the challenge of sphincter-preservation surgery for cancer of the distal 2 cm of the rectum. *International Journal of Radiation Oncology, Biology, Physics* **40**, 569–74.

Morris M, Eifel PJ, Lu J, Grigsby PW, Levenback C, Stevens RE, Rotman M, Gershenson DM & Mutch DG (1999). Pelvic radiation with concurrent chemotherapy compared with pelvic and para-aortic radiation for high-risk cervical cancer. *New England Journal of Medicine* **340**, 1137–43.

Nigro ND, Vaitkevicius VK & Considine B Jr (1993). Combined therapy for cancer of the anal canal: a preliminary report. 1974 [classical article]. *Diseases of the Colon & Rectum* **36**, 709–11.

Northover JM (1991). Epidermoid cancer of the anus – the surgeon retreats [editorial; comment]. *Journal of the Royal Society of Medicine* **84**, 389–90.

O'Connell MJ, Martenson JA, Wieand HS, Krook JE, Macdonald JS, Haller DG, Mayer RJ, Gunderson LL & Rich TA (1994). Improving adjuvant therapy for rectal cancer by combining protracted-infusion fluorouracil with radiation therapy after curative surgery. *New England Journal of Medicine* **331**, 502–7.

Papillon J, Mayer M, Montbarbon JF, Gerard JP, Chassard JL & Bailly C (1983). A new approach to the management of epidermoid carcinoma of the anal canal. *Cancer* **51**, 1830–7.

Rich TA, Skibber JM, Ajani JA, Buchholz DJ, Cleary KR, Dubrow RA, Levin Lynch PM, Meterissian SH & Roubein LD (1995) Preoperative infusional chemoradiation therapy for stage T3 rectal cancer. *International Journal of Radiation Oncology, Biology, Physics* **32**, 1025–9.

Scott N, Hale A, Deakin M, Hand P, Adab FA, Hall C, Williams GT & Elder JB (1998). A histopathological assessment of the response of rectal adenocarcinoma to combination chemo-radiotherapy: relationship to apoptotic activity, p53 and bcl-2 expression. *European Journal of Surgical Oncology* **24**, 169–73.

Sebag-Montefiore, D & Glynne-Jones R (1997). Chemoradiotherapy for rectal cancer – high compliance, low toxicity and early results. *British Journal of Cancer* **76**, 31–31.

Steele RJC & Sebag-Montefiore D (2000). Adjuvant radiotherapy for rectal cancer. *British Journal of Surgery* **86**, 1233–4.

Tobin RL, Mohiuddin M & Marks G (1991). Preoperative irradiation for cancer of the rectum with extrarectal fixation. *International Journal of Radiation Oncology, Biology, Physics* **21**, 1127–32.

Valentini V, Coco C, Cellini N, Picciocchi A, Rosetto ME, Mantini G, Marmirolli L, Barbaro B, Cogliandolo, S, Nuzzo G, Tedesco M, Ambesi-Impiombato F, Cosimelli M & Rotman M (1999a). Preoperative chemoradiotherapy with cisplatin and 5fluorouracil for extraperitoneal T3 rectal cancer: acute toxicity, tumour response, sphincter preservation. *International Journal of Radiation Oncology, Biology, Physics* **45**, 1175–84.

Valentini V, Morganti AG, Fiorentino G, Luzi S, Smaniotto D, Turriziani A, Ratto C, Sofo L, Doglietto GB & Cellini N (1999b). Chemoradiation with raltitrexed ('Tomudex') and concomitant preoperative radiotherapy has potential in the treatment of stage II/III resectable rectal cancer. *Proceedings of the American Society of Clinical Oncology* **18**, 257a.

Wagman R, Minsky BD, Cohen AM, Guillem JG & Paty PP (1998) Sphincter preservation in rectal cancer with preoperative radiation therapy and coloanal anastomosis: long term follow-up. *International Journal of Radiation Oncology, Biology, Physics* **42**, 51–7.

Walsh TN, Noonan N, Hollywood D, Kelly A, Keeling N & Hennessy TP (1996) A comparison of multimodal therapy and surgery for esophageal adenocarcinoma. *New England Journal of Medicine* **335**, 462–7.

Chapter 9

Evidence-based surgery: the synthesis and application of surgical research evidence in the management of rectal cancer

James S McCourtney and John MA Northover

Introduction

Although we might hope that the evidence-based approach would have been the bedrock for the evolution of treatment in any sphere, the extent and nature of that evidence base is not always luminously apparent. Dogma and case load-based experience and attitudes have had a large part to play in the evolution of rectal cancer surgery. The most objective tool, the randomised control trial, has played little part in this very technical surgical area. Considerable debate surrounds many important issues, largely due to the paucity of robust scientific studies carried out to date. This chapter will reflect on the historical development of rectal cancer surgery, going on to debate some, although not all, of the more controversial issues of recent years.

Historical development of surgical technique in rectal cancer

Rectal cancer surgery before the twentieth century was dangerous, and was aimed mainly at those with advanced mechanical complications. In 1908, Ernest Miles described the first Halstedian procedure, abdominoperineal excision, seeking to excise the tumour and its lymphatic drainage, with cure as the target (Miles 1908).

Granshaw has provided us with a clear account of the key developments in this field (Granshaw 1985). Miles' procedure was a combined abdominal and perineal operation, taking particular care to excise the 'zone of upward spread', necessitating a permanent colostomy. Since recurrence could only be prevented by radical excision of the entire rectum, anal canal and sphincters, a large amount of the levatores ani muscles, the contents of the ischiorectal fossae and the bulk of the sigmoid and mesocolon with associated lymphovascular structures, the Miles operation was a considerable undertaking. Other surgeons were not convinced of the need for this degree of surgical invasion, and were unimpressed by Miles' 40 per cent operative mortality. Nevertheless, Miles was able to decrease his local recurrence rate from 54/57 cases operated on via an exclusively perineal approach, to 0/26, treated in 1910 by the abdominoperineal procedure. He reported that the operation was 'virtually bloodless' after dividing the inferior mesenteric artery, and took him just 75–90 minutes to complete. Surgeons gradually moved towards his position, although performance of most of the dissection perineally, avoiding extensive laparotomy and diminishing the risks of surgical shock and sepsis, remained prevalent for several decades. Such an approach, the 'perineoabdominal excision', was devised and used by Gabriel at St Mark's. It comprised extraperitoneal perineal resection of the rectum followed by subsequent limited abdominal surgery to deal with the lymphovascular structures. However, it failed to rival Miles' operation in popularity, despite being shown to be a very safe procedure.

Surgeons at St Mark's Hospital tried to reserve surgery for the most favourable cases, Lockhart-Mummery devising a clinical classification (A, B and C cases) as a guide to potential operability (Lockhart-Mummery 1927). His pathologist colleague, Cuthbert Dukes, compared this clinical grading with the findings in the pathological surgical specimen, concluding that the surgeons were generally too optimistic in their assessment, the tumour usually having progressed more than they surmised. This led to Dukes' development of the first pathological staging system, allowing the first attempts at prognostication, and based on 'scientific' observation (Dukes 1929, 1932). Remarkably Dukes' original staging system has survived all the vicissitudes of the rest of the twentieth century to form the cornerstone of prognostication at the beginning of the current century, although surgeons and pathologists have often found the concept and application of staging difficult, controversial and sometimes confusing (Kyriakos 1986).

Dukes' work with the surgical specimens delivered to him by his surgical colleagues in ever-increasing numbers led him to develop a view of the natural history of the lymphatic drainage of the rectum which was to alter the approach to radical rectal cancer surgery (Dukes 1929, 1940). He carried out meticulous dissections, mapping all lymph glands, involved or not, allowing him to chart 'the exact course and sequence of carcinomatous spread'. This was to provide an objective basis for the move away from the 'necessity' of total rectal excision in some cases: as the lymphatic drainage appeared to be predominantly upwards, rather than in all directions as assumed by Miles, performing a restorative procedure, the 'anterior resection', in which the tumour bearing segment was resected and an anastomosis fashioned, was viewed as a possibility in high-lying rectal and rectosigmoid tumours. Described by Claude Dixon of the Mayo Clinic in the late 1930s, anterior resection was regarded almost as heresy by surgeons who were by then only just accepting Miles' operation as the basis of rectal cancer surgery. The treatment of rectal cancer without excising the anal canal was slow to gain acceptance, and, even in specialist centres, it was not until the 1970s that anterior resection became the operation of choice in the majority of operable cases (Figure 9.1). It reached that stage through the development of a large case load, and the gradual recognition by surgeons that the procedure was as safe as abdominoperineal excision if applied to the 'correct' case. Although the comparison of the novel procedure of anterior resection with the standard abdominoperineal

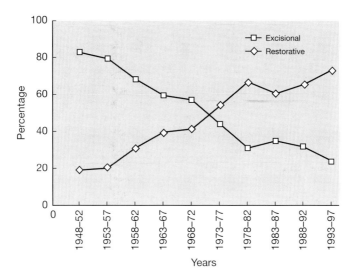

Figure 9.1 Changing trend of restorative and excisional procedures for rectal cancer at St Mark's Hospital, 1948–1997

excision might seem the classic surgical question, there has never been a randomised trial to test this point. As late as the 1980s non-randomised comparisons were being performed and published. Attempts were made to compare outcomes in the same institutions using historical 'controls', or to compare surgical and oncological results between institutions using different policies (Williams *et al.* 1985). By the time these studies were being published, some 50 years after the introduction of anterior resection, the die had been cast, but the very fact of their presentation in the mid 1980s is an indication of the paucity of formal data on the subject, and perhaps the perception of the need for at least some form of scientific comparison. Williams indicated that anterior resection in the late 1970s to early 1980s was attended by a local recurrence rate of 14 per cent compared to 19 per cent for abdominoperineal excision. Such studies, fraught with the biases relating to inter-institutional and historical comparisons, nevertheless concluded the issue to the satisfaction of most surgeons, leaving the ground open for less fundamental issues in rectal cancer surgery.

A quiet but fundamental 'Soviet revolution' began in the late 1960s when the first Russian circular stapling gun was introduced (Fain *et al.* 1975), with a dramatic impact on anastomotic technique. Corroborative data from Goligher and colleagues (1979), as well as Heald in Basingstoke (Heald 1980), paved the way for most surgeons to have the potential technical ability to construct ever lower sphincter-sparing anastomoses. With refinement of stapling techniques the treatment of carcinoma of the lower two thirds of the rectum has been dramatically altered, with far fewer patients now requiring permanent colostomy formation. This development of lower anastomoses, performed in most hospitals across the UK as well as in other countries, was predicated on the acceptance of sphincter-saving surgery based on a small body of science and an ever expanding case load. It will be argued below that this process, the craft-based rather than science-based approach, is the model which surgeons in this field have come to know and love, with randomised trials likely to remain few and far between.

Some key issues in modern rectal cancer surgery

This section does not aim to be comprehensive; rather it seeks to illustrate the range of difficult practical problems faced by surgeons and their fellow travellers in the management of rectal cancer, and some of the methods used in seeking to elucidate them. We will discuss the currently topical question of the possible effects of surgeon-related variables in cancer outcomes; the role of luminal shed cancer cells in local recurrence; and the upper and lower anatomical limits of radical rectal cancer resection.

Surgeon-related variables

Surgeons face the prospect of becoming individually more accountable for the outcome of their efforts in the treatment of many conditions besides rectal cancer. Nevertheless, this condition illustrates some of the difficulties in assessing and acting upon evidence of surgeon-related variables. It cannot be assumed that a 'dose of surgery' is as definable and reproducible as a dose of a particular medicament. Intermingled within this issue there are several phenomena which will modify the outcome in the individual surgeon's practice. These include the surgeon's innate ability, the case mix presented to the surgeon, the volume of cases seen and the training and declared specialty interest of the surgeon. Not all of these are easily controlled either by the surgeon or by those managing a cancer service.

It is perhaps surprising that the importance of who operates has not always been at the forefront of the search for enhanced outcomes in cancer care, although this issue is potentially explosive, addressing as it does the potential comparison of individual surgeons, perhaps on a regular and on an institutionalised basis.

Several studies have looked at the results of individual surgeons, at the effects of volume and case mix, and at the role of specialisation in outcome of surgery for rectal cancer. In an effort to assess the impact of the individual surgeon on the outcome of colorectal cancer surgery, McArdle & Hole (1991) looked at 1128 patients under the care of 15 consultant general surgeons, none of whom declared a specific interest in coloproctology. The results obtained by each surgeon were compared with the others combined. In this way the relative hazard ratio as a measure of outcome was obtained. This effectively indicated time-specific mortality for the selected surgeon against all the other surgeons in the study combined. A value greater than 1 indicated a higher than average mortality. For curative resections the hazard ratios varied amongst surgeons from 0.54–1.46, and for palliative resection from 0.32–1.57. The study concluded that some surgeons perform less than optimal surgery, some are less technically skilled than their counterparts and some surgeons do not provide adequate supervision of trainee surgeons.

Whilst these data were likely to be subject to historical and other biases, a subsequent study by the same group prospectively collected outcome data between 1991 and 1994 on over 3,000 patients presenting to 12 hospitals and 57 surgeons in Central Scotland (McArdle *et al.* 1996). Unfortunately, differences in both case mix and outcome persisted. One of the 12 hospitals had almost double the failure rate of the others. When individual consultants were examined it also appeared that several surgeons were performing less well, even allowing for data adjustment for case mix.

Several studies have assessed immediate outcome following colorectal cancer surgery (Fielding *et al.* 1980; Phillips *et al.* 1984b; McArdle & Hole 1991; Dunn & Fowler 1992; Lothian and Borders Large Bowel Cancer Project 1995; Hermanek & Hohenberger 1996). The results in all have been broadly similar. The St Mary's Large Bowel Cancer Project (Phillips *et al.* 1984a) suggested that the experience of the operator was directly linked to the mortality, length of hospital stay, anastomotic leak rates, blood transfusion requirements, local recurrence of the disease and overall survival.

In the Lothian and Borders Large Bowel Cancer Project, 251 patients (96.5 per cent) with rectal cancer underwent rectal resection, of whom 179 (71.3 per cent) had an anastomosis fashioned (Lothian and Borders Large Bowel Cancer Project 1995). Five of the 28 participating surgeons were responsible for half of these patients. While patients treated by these five surgeons were no more likely to have an anastomosis fashioned, in those where an anastomosis was performed it was much less likely to leak if created by one of these five rather than the remaining 23 participants.

Interpretation of such data carries inherent problems. For example, a surgeon's perception of whether an operation was curative or palliative may influence survival rates in these categories, making the surgeon's data better or worse than average. Likewise, variations in outcome may reflect not only differences amongst surgeons but also variability in the quality of pathological reporting. Stage migration might therefore influence expectation and outcome (Feinstein *et al.* 1985).

Volume of workload and the issue of specialisation are also important considerations when assessing the results of individual surgeons. The effect of volume on outcome of colorectal cancer surgery is, as yet, unproven. Although volume has been shown to be important in coronary artery bypass (Showstack *et al.* 1987) and aortic aneurysm repair (Hannan *et al.* 1992), the effect of volume on outcome following gastrointestinal cancer surgery is not as well established (Jahault 1996). In the Colorectal Cancer Audit of the Royal College of Surgeons there was no evidence that volume had any effect on short-term results, recurrence rates at one year, or on survival rates (Steele 1996). In the Lothian and Borders Large Bowel Cancer Project (1995), the five consultants who performed 50 per cent of all the rectal cancer procedures did have significantly lower anastomotic leak rates, but this in itself could have been a reflection of specialisation rather than volume of cases. Finally, there were no differences in local recurrence rates following rectal cancer surgery performed by 'low volume' surgeons (less than 15 cancers in the study period) compared with the results of high volume surgeons (Hermanek & Hohenberger 1996). As McArdle and colleagues have pointed out, it would at present be misguided to place too much emphasis on volume of workload per se (McArdle *et al.* 1997). With minimal workload levels set in order to qualify as a Cancer Unit (1997), the great worry is that some highly skilled pelvic or gastrointestinal surgeons would be prevented from performing colorectal cancer surgery when instead they should actually be actively encouraged to perform more resections.

Any connection between surgeon specialisation and outcome of rectal cancer surgery is complex. The relatively small numbers of cases treated by any individual surgeon make meaningful statistical analysis difficult. In some studies there was no evidence that more experienced surgeons did better in terms of lower recurrence rates and improved survival when compared with junior counterparts, although the results were not adjusted for case mix (Phillips *et al.* 1984a). Surgery for rectal cancer is acknowledged as being technically more demanding than colonic surgery. It is therefore interesting to note that in the Trent/Wales Audit, whilst numerous nonspecialist surgeons dealing with colonic cancer had excellent results for small numbers of cases, the local recurrence rates following potentially curative resection for rectal cancer were significantly superior for those surgeons who declared a specialist interest (Steele 1996). Other studies (Lockhart-Mummery *et al.* 1976; Whittaker & Goligher 1976; McDermott *et al.* 1981; Jones & Thomson 1982) have supported the role of specialised units in rectal cancer surgery.

Thus, differences in outcome amongst surgeons treating rectal cancer do appear to exist, and indeed may be greater than any additional effect produced by the use of adjuvant chemo- and radiotherapy. The persisting and significant differences in outcome amongst surgeons operating on colorectal cancer strongly support the tenet that this type of surgery should be undertaken by designated specialists. Whether and how evidence on the performance of individual surgeons might be collected and assessed in the future is a challenge yet to be faced by government, representative bodies and each surgeon practising in the field.

Luminally shed cells and local recurrence

Prevention of local recurrence is a key element of rectal cancer surgery. Most local recurrences develop outside the lumen, rather than in the anastomosis; nevertheless, for several decades the identification of luminally shed cells, and their eradication, has been a subject for research and modifications in surgical technique.

A step in minimising risk of local recurrence is held to be cytocidal irrigation of the rectal remnant below the anastomosis. This is achieved by cross-clamping the bowel below the tumour, irrigating below the clamp, followed by division of the cleansed bowel prior to anastomosis. Senior surgeons talk of the higher anastomotic recurrence rates prior to the regular use of rectal stump washout, but there are no formal randomised comparisons of this procedure. The nearest to objective evidence in this issue is the demonstration of the presence of viable cancer cells in the rectal lumen and in the peritoneal cavity outside the anastomosis (Umpleby *et al.* 1984a; Leather *et al.* 1991). The efficacy of various irrigants has been compared to add objectivity to this choice. Colorectal cancer cells are killed as effectively in vitro by chlorhexidine, cetrimide, mercuric perchloride and povidone iodine, while water is ineffective (Umpleby & Williamson 1984b). Mercuric perchloride is probably the most effective cytocidal washout agent in rectal cancer surgery, since blood markedly reduces the efficacy of povidone iodine and chlorhexidine/cetrimide (Docherty *et al.* 1995).

On the evidence available, controversy persists over the need to take steps to irrigate the rectal stump with cytocidal solutions before anastomosis. Most British surgeons irrigate, while most North American surgeons choose not to do so. Even committed adherents of cytocidal washout concede that, in cases where they perform transanal local excision, all the theoretical risks of tumour cell implantation are ignored.

Inferior mesenteric artery division – high versus low tie

It is perhaps remarkable that a debate has persisted concerning whether or not to perform a resection of the proximal centimetre of the inferior mesenteric artery (IMA) and its surrounding tissues. The controversy over the level of lymphovascular division has persisted since Miles recommended division of the IMA just distal to the left colic branch with en bloc removal of distal nodes and bowel (Miles 1908). In the same year, Moynihan promoted the high tie, arguing that the IMA should be ligated and divided flush with the aorta in an effort to remove even more proximal lymph nodes (Moynihan 1908). Dukes showed that the lymphatic spread of cancer ran closely alongside the IMA to its origin at the aorta (Gordon-Watson & Dukes 1930), while evidence from high tie specimens revealed involved nodes proximal to the left colic artery (Gabriel *et al.* 1935). Studies of relatively inferior survival in cases with 'apical node' involvement further strengthened the high tie argument (Gabriel *et al.* 1935). Others have argued that the more radical high tie procedure could downstage a case (from stage C2 to C1), without actually altering the true prognosis, by including in the surgical specimen uninvolved lymph nodes immediately above the site of nodal spread (Morgan 1959).

Critics of the high tie technique have argued that it can threaten the proximal blood supply of the anastomosis which can cause a number of complications which may ultimately require further, more extensive, surgery, although a recent careful study of oxygen saturations in the two procedures did not support the need to preserve the left colic artery by low-tying the IMA (Hall *et al.* 1995). A clinical outcome study, looking at anastomotic leak rates, came to the same conclusion (Corder *et al.* 1995). In non-randomised studies which have compared high and low tie in rectal cancer surgery, no survival benefit has been found (Pezim & Nicholls 1984; Surtees *et al.* 1990). High tie should therefore be employed for technical rather than for oncological reasons, or to promote perfusion; by mobilising the splenic flexure and performing a high tie of the IMA the descending colon is able to reach the anus without tension and with adequate blood supply from the marginal artery.

Total mesorectal excision (TME)

Perhaps the hottest topic in rectal cancer surgery in the past decade, and for the beginning of the new century, concerns the role of total mesorectal excision (TME). TME has been promoted by Heald and his disciples as the surgical treatment of choice for all rectal cancers above 4 cm from the anal verge (MacFarlane *et al.* 1993). The technique is described in detail in standard colorectal surgical texts (Heald 1993; Corman 1999; Keighley & Williams 1999). The Basingstoke data have been independently analysed by MacFarlane and colleagues, looking at results over the period 1978–1991 (MacFarlane *et al.* 1993). The actuarial local recurrence rate after curative anterior resection was 4 per cent at five years and the overall recurrence rate was 18 per cent. For ten year follow-up the corresponding figures were 4 per cent and 19 per cent.

However, 'total mesorectal confusion' has come about due to the ambiguity of the word 'total'. Heald's original description of the operation promulgated both the removal of the whole *length* of the mesorectum and the maintenance of the integrity of the mesorectum within its fascial envelope (its radial *breadth*). Over the subsequent two decades, surgeons have argued about the relative roles of these two aspects of the meaning of 'total':

- Many surgeons argue that in the radial sense – preserving the mesorectum within its fascia – they have always adhered to dissection in the plane outside the mesorectal fascia (Heald's 'holy plane') Figure 9.2 (Heald 1993), and that Heald has merely emphasised good practice rather than contributing a new idea.
- There has also been argument that in its longitudinal sense, total mesorectal excision is new – a move towards increased radicality from accepted practice in sphincter-saving rectal cancer resection – and that its place is not proven.

Based on the development of our understanding of the anatomy of rectal lymphatic drainage over the past 70 years, from Dukes onward, and based on the precepts of Halsted, rectal surgeons have accepted that the mesorectum should be kept intact within its envelope. Having said that, it has to be conceded to Heald that standard surgical texts have not emphasised this in their descriptions of anterior resection; indeed, just as Goligher's text, of almost Biblical influence in decades past, depicted the mesorectum as a vestigial postrectal strip, so too do we find an almost identical

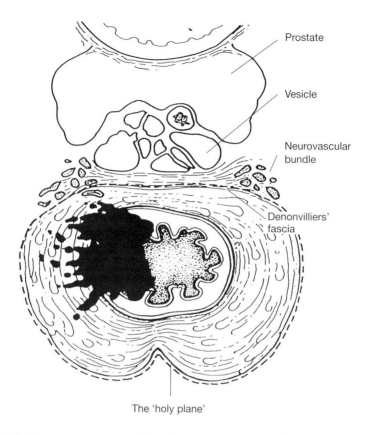

Prostate

Vesicle

Neurovascular bundle

Denonvilliers' fascia

The 'holy plane'

Figure 9.2 The mesorectum and its radial resection plane (from Rob & Smith's *Operative Surgery*, Heald 1993)

rendition in the Keighley & Williams equivalent text today (Goligher 1984; Keighley & Williams 1999). Thus Heald's promotion of appropriate radial dissection must be commended, and has certainly led to more surgeons performing this part of rectal cancer dissection better. His insistence on precise sharp dissection under vision can be contrasted with the continued promulgation of blunt dissection using the whole hand, still seen in Rob & Smith's textbook, perhaps the leading atlas of surgical technique (Murray & Veidenheimer 1993). (Figure 9.3).

In Scandinavia TME has been embraced by many surgeons. The data from the population-based study at Linkoping compared results for rectal cancer surgery in three surgical departments over the periods 1984–1986 (group 1) and 1990–1992 (group 2) (Arbman *et al.* 1996). During the latter period they adopted the technique of TME. In group 1, 134 patients had undergone either curative anterior resection or APER. In group 2, 128 curative TMEs were performed. There were no differences between the groups in terms of tumour stage, rate of curative surgery or postoperative

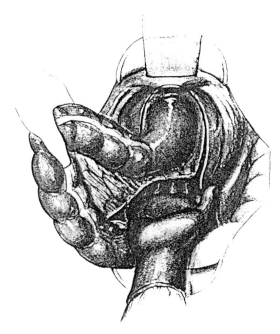

Figure 9.3 Blunt dissection of the rectum in the 1990s (from Rob & Smith's *Operative Surgery*, Murray and Veidenheimer 1993)

morbidity and mortality. Actuarial analysis showed a significant reduction in local recurrence rates and increase in crude survival at four years in group 2 compared with group 1. However, in this study there was a significant decrease in local recurrence after APER following the adoption of TME. Given that APER by definition should incorporate TME, such data could strengthen the argument that more meticulous dissection in the extrafascial 'holy plane' was the key component in reducing local recurrence rates in rectal cancer surgery in Linkoping, rather than the perhaps unnecessarily radical TME with its associated increased risk of morbidity (Scholefield & Northover 1995).

In a review from the Sloane Kettering Cancer Center a local recurrence rate of 7.3 per cent was found in a consecutive series of 246 patients with rectal cancer treated by TME. This series included curative and palliative resections. The authors concluded that this was a superior local recurrence rate to that previously obtained when they used a combination of conventional surgery and combined modality adjuvant therapy (Enker *et al.* 1995).

In an analysis of local recurrence rates after surgery for rectal cancer, McCall and colleagues found a median local recurrence rate of 18.5 per cent after follow-up in 10,465 patients. Of the subgroup of 1033 patients who had undergone TME the local recurrence rate was 7.1 per cent (McCall *et al.* 1995).

One particular drawback with TME is the high rate of anastomotic dehiscence. In the Basingstoke data reported in 1994 there was a major anastomotic leak rate of 11 per cent in 219 patients undergoing low anterior resection with TME. A further 6.4 per cent of asymptomatic leaks were noted on contrast enemas. TME may result in a denuded and relatively devascularised anorectal remnant. A routine defunctioning stoma is therefore recommended when TME is performed (Karanjia *et al.* 1991).

The morbidity associated with TME has led some surgeons to adopt a selective policy. In a consecutive series of patients referred to a single surgeon in Edinburgh, Scotland a policy of subtotal mesorectal excision (SME) (distal margin excised 5 cm below the tumour) was used for all rectal cancers except those where the lower border of the tumour was 7–8 cm from the anal verge (Aitken 1996). Sixty-four patients underwent curative resection. In 30 patients followed-up at a mean of 30 months there were no isolated pelvic or anastomotic recurrences although four (13 per cent) developed distant recurrence. The cumulative recurrence-free survival rate at 24 months was 84 per cent. Aitken argued that his SME policy produced a similar result to that of TME because studies (Gilchrist & David 1938; Grinnell 1942, 1966; Dukes 1943) have shown that retrograde tumour metastases in the mesorectum were normally within 2 cm and rarely more than 5 cm from the lower border of the tumour. More recent work has shown distal deposits in 4 of 20 patients 1–3 cm below the tumour (Scott *et al.* 1995) and 12 of 50 patients 2–5 cm below the tumour (Reynolds *et al.* 1996). It is also worthy of note that in 1982 Heald and colleagues reported the practice of dividing the mesorectum at least 5 cm below the tumour for selected upper rectal cancer, whilst still achieving very low local recurrence rates (Heald *et al.* 1982). This practice was still used by the Basingstoke group as recently as 1994 (Karanjia *et al.* 1994).

In a series from Gateshead in the North East of England potentially curative TME was performed in only 59 per cent of patients presenting with rectal or rectosigmoid cancer (Hainsworth *et al.* 1997). Of these, 12 of 45 patients had TME performed for upper third or rectosigmoid tumours. This controversial application of TME yielded a local recurrence rate of 11 per cent and an anastomotic leak rate of 16 per cent. Those authors questioned the role of TME for curative resection of upper third tumours.

Currently many surgeons would perform SME when faced with an upper third rectal or rectosigmoid cancer. However, given the data above relating to distal satellite deposits of tumour in the mesorectum they would all perform quite an extensive distal clearance of mesentery in the region of 5 cm, making the anastomosis at the level of the junction of mid and lower third of rectum. The current debate on the role of TME in upper third rectal cancer has mirrored the debate in gastric cancer surgery – total gastrectomie de principale versus total gastrectomie de necessitaire (Phillips 1998). Whether TME should always be performed in all cases of rectal cancer or instead only in certain circumstances will require a multicentre, prospective randomised trial comparing local recurrence, five-year survival rate, functional outcome and associated complications (Carter 1997; Hainsworth *et al.* 1997).

The notion of longitudinal TME for all cases is without a sound evidence base. That excellent local recurrence rates can be achieved through its use does not compensate for the functional and morbidity deficit which can occur as a result of the removal of too much normal rectum below a mid or high rectal cancer. A protocol to compare TME and shorter resection in mid and high rectal cancers may launch as a multicentre randomised controlled trial in the near future.

Summary

Rectal cancer surgery is a very good example of the craft-based approach to evolution of technique. Scientific observation has played a significant part, but the randomised trial has been secondary to individual experience and the building of opinion based on case load. Although randomised trials are in progress in several rectal cancer surgery fields, we predict that the time-honoured methods will mainly determine the role of newer techniques, such as laparoscopic rectal cancer surgery.

References

Aitken RJ (1996). Mesorectal excision for rectal cancer. *British Journal of Surgery* **83**, 214–16.

Arbman G. *et al.* (1996). Local recurrence following total mesorectal excision for rectal cancer. *British Journal of Surgery* **83**, 375–79.

Carter P (1997). Evaluation of a policy of total mesorectal excision for rectal and rectosigmoid tumours (letter). *British Journal of Surgery* **84**, 1749.

Corder A *et al.* (1995). Flush aortic tie versus selective preservation of the ascending left colic artery in low anterior resection for rectal carcinoma. *British Journal of Surgery* **79**, 680–82.

Corman ML (ed.) (1999). Carcinoma of the rectum. *Colon Rectal Surgery.* Philadelphia, Lippincott Raven: pp 786–89.

Docherty JG *et al.* (1995). Efficacy of tumouricidal agents in vitro and in vivo. *British Journal of Surgery* **82**, 1050–52.

Dukes C (1929). The spread of cancer of the rectum. *British Journal of Surgery* **17**, 643–48.

Dukes C (1932). The classification of cancer of the rectum. *Journal of Pathology and Bacteriology* **35**, 323–32.

Dukes C (1940). Cancer of the rectum: an analysis of 1,000 cases. *Journal of Pathology and Bacteriology* **50**, 527.

Dukes CE (1943). The surgical pathology of rectal cancer. *Proceedings of the Royal Society of Medicine* **37**, 131–44.

Dunn DC & Fowler S (1992). Comparative audit: an experimental study of 147,882 general surgical admissions during 1990. *British Journal of Surgery* **79**, 1073–76.

Enker W *et al.* (1995). Total mesorectal excision in the operative treatment of carcinoma of the rectum. *Journal of the American College of Surgeons* **181**, 335–46.

Fain S *et al.* (1975). Use of mechanical suturing apparatus in low colorectal anastomosis. *Archives of Surgery* **110**.

Feinstein A *et al.* (1985). Stage migration and new diagnostic techniques as a source of misleading statistics for survival in cancer. *New England Journal of Medicine* **312**, 1604–08.

Fielding LP *et al.* (1980). Anastomotic integrity after operations for large-bowel cancer: a multicentre study. *British Medical Journal* **281**.

Gabriel W *et al.* (1935). Lymphatic spread in cancer of the rectum. *British Journal of Surgery* **23**, 395–413.

Gilchrist RK & David VC (1938). Lymphatic spread of carcinoma of the rectum. *Annals of Surgery* **108**, 621–42.

Goligher J (1984). *Surgery of the Anus, Rectum and Colon.* London, Balliere Tindall.

Goligher J C *et al.* (1979). Experience with the Russian model 249 suture gun for anastomosis of the rectum. *Surgery Gynecology and Obstetrics* **148**, 517–24.

Gordon-Watson C & Dukes C (1930). The treatment of carcinoma of the rectum with radium with an introduction on the spread of cancer of the rectum. *British Journal of Surgery* **17**, 643–69.

Granshaw L (1985). *St Mark's Hospital, London. A social history of a specialist hospital,* King Edward's Hospital Fund for London.

Grinnell RS (1942). The lymphatic and venous spread of carcinoma of the rectum. *Annals of Surgery* **116**, 200–16.

Grinnell RS (1966). Lymphatic block with atypical and retrograde lymphatic metastasis and spread of carcinoma of the colon and rectum. *Annals of Surgery* **163**, 272–80.

Hainsworth PJ *et al.* (1997). Evaluation of a policy of total mesorectal excision for rectal and rectosigmoid cancers. *British Journal of Surgery* **84**, 652–56.

Hall NP *et al.* (1995). High tie of the inferior mesenteric artery in distal colorectal resections – a safe vascular procedure. *International Journal of Colorectal Disease* **10**, 29–32.

Hannan EL *et al.* (1992). A longitudinal analysis of the relationships between in-hospital mortality in New York state and the volume of abdominal aortic aneurysm surgeries performed. *Health Services Research* **27**, 517–42.

Heald R (1993). Anterior resection of the rectum. *Rob & Smith's Operative Surgery: Surgery of the Colon, Rectum and Anus.* L. Fielding and S. Goldberg. Oxford, Butterworth-Heinemann: 456–71.

Heald R *et al.* (1982). The mesorectum in rectal cancer surgery – the clue to pelvic recurrence? *British Journal of Surgery.* **69**, 613–16.

Heald RJ (1980). Towards fewer colostomies: the impact of circular stapling devices on the surgery of rectal cancer in a district hospital. *British Journal of Surgery* **60**, 198–200.

Hermanek P & Hohenberger W (1996). The importance of volume in colorectal cancer surgery. *European Journal of Surgical Oncology* **22**(3), 213–5.

Jahault J (1996). The importance of volume for outcome in cancer surgery – an overview. *European Journal of Surgical Oncology* **22**, 205–15.

Jones PF & Thomson HJ (1982). Long term results of a consistent policy of sphincter preservation in the treatment of carcinoma of the rectum. *British Journal of Surgery* **69**, 564–68.

Karanjia N *et al.* (1994). Leakage from stapled low anastomosis after total mesorectal excision for carcinoma of the rectum. *British Journal of Surgery* **81**, 1224–26.

Karanjia ND *et al.* (1991). Risk of peritonitis and fatal septicaemia and the need to defunction the low anastomosis. *British Journal of Surgery* **78**, 196–98.

Keighley MRB & Williams NS eds. (1999). *Surgery of the Anus, Rectum and Colon.* London, W. B. Saunders.

Kyriakos M (1986). The President's cancer, the Dukes classification, and confusion. *Archives of Pathological Laboratory Medicine* **109**, 1063–66.

Leather AJM *et al.* (1991). Passage of shed intraluminal colorectal cancer cells across a sealed anastomosis. *British Journal of Surgery* **78**, 756.

Lockhart-Mummery HE *et al.* (1976). The results of surgical treatment for carcinoma of the rectum at St Mark's Hospital from 1948 to 1972. *British Journal of Surgery* **63**, 673–77.

Lockhart-Mummery J (1927). Two hundred cases of cancer of the rectum treated by perineal excision. *British Journal of Surgery* **14**, 110–24.

Lothian and Borders Large Bowel Cancer Project (1995). Lothian and Borders large bowel cancer project 1995. Immediate outcome after surgery. *British Journal of Surgery* **82**, 888–90.

MacFarlane JK *et al.* (1993). Mesorectal excision for rectal cancer. *The Lancet* **i**, 457–60.

McArdle CS & Hole D (1991). Impact of variability among surgeons on postoperative morbidity and mobility and ultimate survival. *British Medical Journal* **302**, 1501–05.

McArdle CS *et al.,* eds. (1997). Outcome following surgery for colorectal cancer. In: *Recent Advances in Surgery.* Edinburgh, Churchill Livingstone.

McArdle CS *et al.* (1996). Colorectal cancer: a continuing problem. *GI Cancer* **1**, 171–76.

McCall J *et al.* (1995). Analysis of local recurrence rates after surgery alone for rectal cancer. *International Journal of Colorectal Disease* **10**, 126–32.

McDermott FT *et al.* (1981). Comparative results of surgical management of single carcinomas of the colon and rectum: a series of 1939 patients managed by one surgeon. *British Journal of Surgery* **68**, 850–55.

Miles W (1908). A method of performing abdominoperineal excision for carcinoma of the rectum and of the terminal portion of the pelvic colon. *The Lancet* , 1812–13.

Morgan CN (1959). The comparative results and treatment for cancer of the rectum. *Postgraduate Medicine* **26**, 135.

Moynihan BGA (1908). The surgical treatment of cancer of the sigmoid flexure and rectum. *Surgery Gynecologoy and Obstetrics* **6**, 463–66.

Murray J & Veidenheimer M (1993). Abdominoperineal excision of the rectum. *Rob & Smith's Operative Surgery: Surgery of the Colon, Rectum and Anus.* L. Fielding and S. Goldberg. Oxford, Butterworth-Heinemann, 472–87.

Pezim M & Nicholls R (1984). Survival after high or low ligation of the inferior mesenteric artery during curative surgery for rectal cancer. *Annals of Surgery* **200**, 729–33.

Phillips RK *et al.* (1984a). Local recurrence following 'curative' surgery for large bowel cancer: I. The overall picture. *British Journal of Surgery* **71**(1), 12–16.

Phillips RK *et al.* (1984b). Local recurrence following curative surgery for large bowel cancer: II The rectum and rectosigmoid. *British Journal of Surgery* **71**, 17–20.

Phillips RKS (1998). Rectal Cancer. *Colorectal Surgery.* R. K. S. Phillips. London, W.B. Saunders, 80–1.

Reynolds J *et al.* (1996). Pathological evidence in support of total mesorectal excision in the management of rectal cancer. *British Journal of Surgery* **83**, 1112–15.

Scholefield J & Northover J (1995). Surgical management of rectal cancer. *British Journal of Surgery* **82**, 745–48.

Scott N *et al.* (1995). Total mesorectal excision and local recurrence: a study of tumour spread in the mesorectum distal to rectal cancer. *British Journal of Surgery* **82**, 1031–33.

Showstack J *et al.* (1987). Association of volume with outcome of coronary artery bypass graft surgery. *Journal of the American Medical Association* **257**, 785–89.

Steele RJC (1996). The influence of surgeon case volume on outcome in site-specific cancer surgery. *European Journal of Surgical Oncology* **22**, 211–13.

Surtees P *et al.* (1990). High versus low ligation of the inferior mesenteric artery in rectal cancer. *British Journal of Surgery* **77**, 618–21.

Umpleby HC *et al.* (1984a). Viability of exfoliated colorectal carcinoma cells. *British Journal of Surgery* **71**, 659–63.

Umpleby UC & Williamson RCN (1984b). The efficacy of agents employed to prevent anastomotic recurrence in colorectal carcinoma. *Annals of the Royal College of Surgeons of England* **66**, 192.

Whittaker M & Goligher JC (1976). The prognosis after surgical treatment for carcinoma of the rectum. *British Journal of Surgery* **63**, 384–88.

Williams N *et al.* (1985). The outcome following sphincter-saving resection and abdomino-perineal resection for low rectal cancer. *British Journal of Surgery* **72**, 595–98.

PART 4

Management of Liver Metastases

Chapter 10

Imaging and biopsy of colorectal liver metastases

Michele M Marshall and John B Karani

Introduction

In patients with colorectal malignancy, the presence of liver metastases is the most accurate predictor of survival. Following apparently curative resection, 50 per cent of patients die within five years, the majority from disseminated disease; hepatic involvement is a feature in 50 per cent of patients (Balfe 1992). Recently, there have been reports of improved survival following partial hepatectomy for liver metastases: five-year survival rates approach 25 per cent in most series and reach 60 per cent for unifocal disease (Adson 1990; Tsao *et al.* 1994; Sugarbaker 1999)

Detection of focal liver lesions pre-operatively is dependent on fundamental differences between normal liver parenchyma and metastases – first, an intrinsic difference in tissue density and cellular components and, second, differences in vascularity and tissue haemodynamics. Current imaging techniques reliably identify metastases greater than 4 cm. However, techniques vary in the type of lesion which they will miss or incorrectly characterise. A focused, multimodality approach will increase the accuracy of lesion detection and staging (Wernecke 1991; Soyer *et al.* 1993). Currently, generally available equipment specifications allow reliable identification of lesions as small as 2 cm, but the detection of these is limited by spatial resolution. Even if detected, the characterisation of lesions less than 1 cm is poor on pre-operative imaging. It is these undetected, subcentimetre lesions which almost always account for the late presentation of disseminated disease (Paul *et al.* 1996).

In order to increase the sensitivity of liver staging we need to examine those cases that apparently have occult hepatic involvement. Three situations can be considered:

- lesions of 1 cm or more which were not detected because of failure of the chosen technique;
- true occult lesions, below the threshold for detection on standard staging imaging;
- missed lesions where in retrospect the lesions were identifiable.

While technological advances and large comparative studies are continuing to improve the accuracy of hepatic staging, the use of currently available resources can be rationalised by employing accepted protocols for the management of patients in specific clinical settings. The aims of imaging, and thus the strategies and techniques used, will vary for patients at their initial presentation, follow-up and when being considered for hepatic resection of metastatic deposits.

Review of current techniques

Ultrasound

Ultrasound provides a rapid, inexpensive, readily available examination. Most hospitals have good-quality equipment with regular upgrade programmes to encompass the rapid developments in ultrasound technology. Ultrasound does not involve ionising radiation and it is accepted that in standard use it has no harmful effects. High-frequency sound is emitted from the transducer, transmitted through the body and reflected at any tissue interface. The same transducer detects the reflections and a picture of the insonated structures is produced using the same principles as RADAR.

During the examination the patient is supine, and a systematic examination of the parenchyma and liver outline is undertaken using an intercostal and subcostal approach. A search for extrahepatic disease, particularly pleural effusions, periportal and coeliac lymph nodes, is also performed. Standard equipment uses tailored settings for abdominal scanning and use electronic curvilinear array transducers with a frequency of 3.5–5 MHz. Colour Doppler ultrasound facilitates examination of the vasculature and portal vein thrombosis, although uncommon in uncomplicated metastatic disease, is easily demonstrated.

Computed tomography

In contrast to conventional x-ray techniques, the development of computed tomography (CT) has allowed characterisation of different soft tissues. A series of images is produced comprising axial slices through the area of interest. When reviewed in sequence, the series enables us to determine the 3-dimensional relationships of internal structures. Conventional CT scanners acquire images slice by slice with a scan time through the liver of approxiamately 1.5 minutes. Helical CT scanners acquire images much more rapidly and the liver can be easily scanned within a single breathold (approximately 15–30 seconds). When considering focal lesions within the liver, it has been shown that lesion conspicuity is greatest in the portal venous phase of enhancement of the liver with iodinated contrast media (Hollett 1995; Kuszyk 1996). Intravenous contrast is administered via a cannula at a rate of 2–3 mls per second (total volume 100 mls) and images subsequently acquired starting just above the dome of the liver during the portal venous phase of enhancement. The development of faster scanners has led to an increase in the sensitivity of CT for detection of focal liver lesions. First, the liver can be examined using thinner-slice thickness, which, although increasing the dose of ionising radiation, leads to much improved spatial resolution such that demonstration of subcentimetre lesions is now possible (Weg *et al.* 1998). Second, shorter scan times mean that misregistration artefacts from breathing are minimised, while also allowing scans to be acquired during the early, arterial phase of hepatic enhancement. Dual-phase helical CT is performed with a breathold technique and rapid infusion of intravenous contrast (100–150 ml at 3 ml/sec). Scans are acquired initially at 25 seconds following the start of the infusion and repeated at 60 seconds producing arterial and portal phase scans. Some authors have shown improved sensitivity for detection of focal lesions with the addition of arterial phase scans, owing to the detection of small, hypervascular lesions not seen on the portal venous phase scans (Hollett 1996). Although of some importance, the benefit from arterial phase scanning in colorectal malignancy is likely to be minimal as hypervascular metastases are rare, while the false positive rate resulting from detection of small haemangiomas would result in excessive investigation in an emotionally charged clinical setting (Ch'en *et al.* 1997).

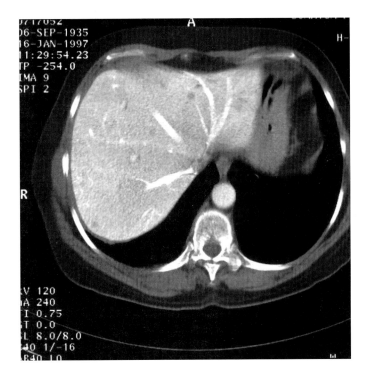

Figure 10.1 Portal venous phase helical CT scan demonstrating several subcentimetre lesions in segments III, IV, VII and VIII

CT arterial portography

CT arterial portography (CTAP) is an invasive technique designed to increase lesion conspicuity on CT scanning. Common femoral arterial puncture is performed and a catheter placed in the superior mesenteric artery (SMA) in the same manner as for indirect portography. The patient is transferred to the CT scanner and intravenous iodinated contrast is infused into the SMA at a rate of 3 ml/sec. Scans are acquired at 45 seconds after the start of the infusion, i.e. during the phase of portal venous enhancement, contrast having reached the liver directly via the portal system. As the liver has not received a prior contrast load (as with conventional dual-phase scanning), any areas of the liver which do not have a portal venous supply will show up as stark contrast to the rest of the liver, which enhances dramatically with the high concentration of contrast delivered.

Magnetic resonance imaging

Magnetic resonance imaging (MRI) uses non-ionising radiation (radiofrequency) within a strong magnetic field. The absorbed energy is released from the cell nuclei in a specific manner proportional to proton density, allowing differentiation of soft tissues. This results in a change in the magnetic field, which is translated into a 'signal' of varying intensity and plotted in a similar way to CT to produce a representation of a slice through the body. Unlike CT, however, the potential exists to display the signals obtained or 'dataset' in any plane, allowing relationships of adjacent structures to be interrogated from various aspects. Different sequences of radio frequency can be used to obtain information about tissue content and several images in one orientation are usually acquired demonstrating different tissue characteristics.

MRI of the liver involves an examination time of approximately 20 minutes. There are some patients who cannot tolerate the claustrophobic conditions during the scan and others in whom MRI is contraindicated due to metal implants, pacemakers, replacement valves or recent surgery. As yet, there have been no harmful effects demonstrated resulting from its use, making sequential scanning an acceptable option. In patients with colorectal cancer, specific sequences are used which enhance lesion conspicuity and demonstrate the relationship of deposits to the hepatic and portal veins when hepatic resection is being considered.

Nuclear medicine

Hepatic perfusion imaging is no longer widely used for detection of metastases, largely because it has been superseded by newer, more accurate techniques. Recent advances in tomographic techniques and the development of radioimmunodetection with radio-labelled monoclonal antibodies as well as positron emission tomography (PET) present an exciting step forward in functional imaging of tumours, although as yet the specificity remains low. While good results have been reported for detection of extrahepatic disease in colorectal cancer patients, the results have not been as good for liver metastases (Divgi *et al.* 1993; Delbeke 1999; Fong *et al.* 1999).

Principles of contrast-enhanced imaging

Identification of a focal hepatic lesion is by virtue of the difference between its intrinsic tissue characteristics and those of the surrounding hepatic parenchyma. The aim of contrast enhanced imaging is to increase sensitivity of the examination by increasing lesion conspicuity. Current techniques that employ contrast agents utilise three fundamental differences in the tissue characteristics of normal liver and metastatic deposits.

Tissue vascularity

The vascular supply to the liver is complex, with approximately two thirds of inflow via the portal vein, the rest from the systemic arterial supply. Since colorectal deposits characteristically are not arterialised but interrupt portal flow, they appear of lower attenuation than the surrounding normal liver in a phase of maximal liver parenchymal enhancement. This can be achieved with any imaging technique by using vascular phase contrast media. Non- ionic iodinated contrast media is used in computed tomography (CT) to increase attenuation of the X-ray beam by tissues that have a good vascular supply and uptake of the contrast medium. Gadolinium salts act in a similar way for magnetic resonance imaging (MRI) by increasing the signal returned from tissues with good contrast uptake. Recent developments in colour Doppler imaging utilise new contrast agents based on microbubbles in solution, measuring between 4–8 microns, which are injected intravenously and are stable for five to ten minutes in the circulation, passing through capillary beds without significant degradation. These simulate red cells and produce an amplified Doppler signal from flowing blood giving increased signal-to-noise ratios. Vascular tumours can be detected using these agents (Bartolozzi *et al.* 1998).

Cellular components

Tissue-specific contrast agents have recently been developed for use in MRI, which have been shown to be of value in imaging focal liver lesions. Super-paramagnetic iron oxides (SPIOs, ferrumoxides) contain iron particles, which are phagocytosed in the liver by Kupffer cells. Following intravenous administration, normal liver parenchyma will return a low signal intensity owing to the accumulation of these iron particles and non liver cell tumours can be identified as areas of absent uptake and a higher signal intensity (Hagspiel *et al.* 1995; Seneterre *et al.* 1996; Ward *et al.* 1999). Levovist, one of the microbubble contrast agents used for Doppler ultrasound, is also cleared by the liver, accumulating in Kupffer cells in the liver parenchyma. Again, with specialised image processing techniques, tumours that are not derived from liver cells may be detected as space-occupying lesions with no contrast uptake (Blomley *et al*. 1999).

Manganese (mangafodipir trisodium, MnDPDP) is a tumour-specific agent metabolised by hepatocytes. It can be used in a similar way to SPIOs, deposits being represented by areas of absent uptake (Figure 10.2), but in addition a hepatocellular tumour will be evident on delayed imaging as an area of focal uptake (Kane *et al.* 1997). Lipiodol has been used in hepatic angiography for hepatocellular carcinoma in a similar way, with CT scanning at 7–10 days when clearance from normal parenchyma will have occurred.

Splanchnic or systemic blood supply

The liver has a unique dual circulation, with reciprocity and balance of arterial and portal flow. Metastases, conversely, retain the characteristics of their tissue of origin and have a predominantly arterial supply (Kan *et al.* 1993). It has been postulated therefore that, as the volume of metastatic deposits increases, the volume of blood flowing to the liver via the hepatic artery increases. Several studies have tried to demonstrate an increase in hepatic arterial flow in patients with colorectal carcinoma and liver metastases. Dynamic hepatic scintigraphy was the first technique to demonstrate this alteration in vascular supply and the hepatic perfusion index has been shown to have a sensitivity equal to current CT and MRI (Leveson *et al.* 1985; Hemingway *et al.* 1992; Carter *et al.* 1996). More recently, Doppler ultrasound has been used to demonstrate the same effect, although the reproducibility of this technique has made validation difficult (Leen *et al.* 1995; Fowler *et al.* 1998; Oppo *et al.* 1998). A further study suggests that the degree of hepatic enhancement on CT during the arterial phase may predict patients who will subsequently develop metastases (Platt *et al.* 1997). Although at an early stage, the importance of these studies should not be ignored. If reproducible methods can be developed, this change in haemodynamics may allow us to detect previously occult infiltration and microscopic metastases. Even with recent improvements in spatial resolution attainable with axial imaging, now in the order of 5 mm, movement artefacts and radiation dose will continue to limit detection of small lesions using conventional techniques.

Is there a gold standard?

As yet, no established pre-operative imaging technique has achieved 100 per cent sensitivity. Histological comparative data are limited to resected lesions and random per-operative liver biopsy. Intra-operative ultrasound is widely used but follow-up studies show this to have a varying sensitivity (Knol *et al.* 1993, Semelka *et al.* 1999), though in general a good specificity. Although many authors have looked at the sensitivity of various imaging techniques over the last 10–15 years, the speed at which radiological techniques and equipment have improved during this time has meant that there are few studies which compare techniques performed to current standards. Along with the improved resolution of ultrasound machines and CT scanners, development of new contrast agents in ultrasound and MRI means that sensitivities of all imaging modalities have increased. Helical contrast-enhanced CT, MRI and CTAP are all comparable in accuracy, with sensitivities between 70 and 88 per cent for MR and CT in recent published series (Zerhouni *et al.* 1996) and an

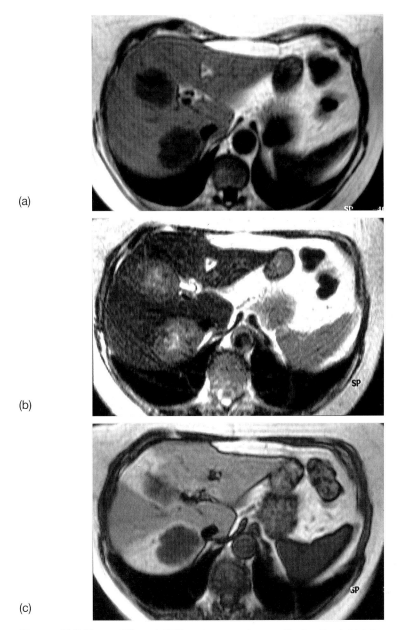

(a)

(b)

(c)

Figure 10.2 Three different MRI sequences in a patient with right lobe metastases
(a) T1 weighted scan shows two large right lobe metastases
(b) T2 weighted scan through the same lesions
(c) T1 weighted MRI following intravenous MnDPDP, a hepatocyte specific agent.
Conspicuity of the deposits is increased owing to accumulation of manganese in
peritumoral sinusoids and a negative-contrast effect reflecting lack of uptake by the
tumour deposits themselves

accepted sensitivity of 100 per cent for lesions greater than 2 cm (Ward *et al.* 1999). Ward *et al.* (ibid.) compared SPIO-enhanced MRI with dual-phase CT and found sensitivities of 99 and 94 per cent, respectively, for lesions greater than 1 cm, although overall sensitivities were 80 and 75 per cent, respectively. In a recent large randomised controlled study, Zerhouni *et al.* (1996) found both helical contrast-enhanced CT and gadolinium-enhanced MRI to have accuracies of 85 per cent. This relatively low figure reflects their study design, which, unlike many previous studies, took the gold standard as no evidence of metastases at CT or MR follow-up between 9 and 15 months after the initial assessment. This provided an additional measure of truth, reflecting the inherent inability to detect microscopic involvement, accounting for sensitivities of CT and MR of 62 and 70 per cent, respectively.

CTAP has the highest sensitivity, but the costs and morbidity associated with this invasive procedure have limited its use. Particularly, despite a high sensitivity, the technique carries a low specificity owing to misinterpretation of flow and movement artefacts (Nelson *et al.* 1992; Valls *et al.* 1998). It offers greatest advantage when considering a patient with metastases for partial hepatectomy, as the detection of additional lesions may alter and even preclude surgical management (Figure 10.3). As experience with newer MR techniques increase however, it is likely that SPIO enhanced MRI and intra-operative ultrasound (IOUS) will provide similar results with less expense and the avoidance of an invasive radiological procedure (Bellin *et al.* 1994; Seneterre *et al.* 1996; Semelka *et al.* 1997). Moreover, it may be considered more acceptable to find an occasional unsuspected lesion rather than deny surgery to a patient on the basis of a false positive finding at CTAP.

Reported series attribute the lowest sensitivities to ultrasound, with sensitivities between 48 and 77 per cent (Wernecke *et al.* 1991; Leen *et al.* 1995; Carter *et al.* 1996). Technological advances have resulted in higher-resolution machines but the cost of upgrading current equipment means these are not as yet widely available. Ultrasound remains, however, a safe, cost-effective investigation and as such provides a good screening examination with accuracies similar to CT and MR for lesions greater than 2 cm.

Which technique?

The design of an imaging algorithm should be specific to the clinical setting, as the requirements are different for a number of patient groups.

Initial presentation

All patients presenting with colorectal cancer can be considered with respect to their primary tumour and to disseminated disease. Between 15 and 30 per cent of patients will have liver metastases at presentation and a proportion of these will have been identified as the presenting feature. However, it is accepted that in almost all circumstances control of local disease by resection of the primary tumour will improve quality of life and it may prolong survival even in the presence of disseminated disease (Sugarbaker 1999).

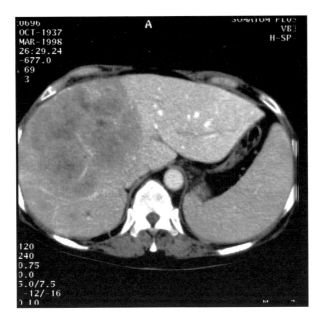

(a)

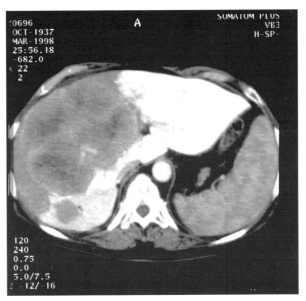

(b)

Figure 10.3

(a) Portal venous phase helical CT scan showing a large right-lobe metastasis and some heterogeneity elsewhere in the right lobe

(b) CTAP results in enhanced conspicuity of a satellite tumour in relation to the dominant metastasis

Imaging is aimed at the detection of metastases prior to the primary resection, so that surgery may be planned as curative or palliative. It is reasonable to advocate ultrasound as an initial screening method, since it may be more readily available and is less invasive. If bilobar metastases are seen on ultrasound, then further pre-operative imaging is unnecessary. The high sensitivity of ultrasound combined with contrast-enhanced CT of the abdomen and pelvis gives an acceptable detection rate for this to be the mainstay of first-line staging of colorectal carcinoma. Whilst it is most unusual to see lung metastases in the absence of liver involvement, a pre-operative CXR provides baseline information and adds little to the radiation burden whilst providing further confirmation of disease status.

If a curative resection is performed, then surveillance scanning is required so that any liver metastases are detected at an early stage and hepatic resection or percutaneous ablation can be considered where disease is limited to the liver.

Oncology setting

Treatment of disseminated disease has been shown to prolong survival. All treatment options are associated with considerable morbidity, and here there is an extended role for imaging. First, we must assess the response of the disease to treatment, usually three months after any treatment programme has been instigated. This may be done with ultrasound, MRI or CT but ultrasound has the disadvantage of being operator-dependent, making direct comparison of scans more difficult. Second, imaging may be required to demonstrate complications of therapy, particularly those consequent to bone marrow suppression.

Having achieved a response, surveillance scanning should continue with three questions in mind:

- Is there evidence of extrahepatic disease?
- Is there disease progression or breakthrough despite continuing therapy?
- Is there disease progression in previously static or eradicated disease?

Hepatobiliary surgery

Current indications for hepatic resection in colorectal cancer are fewer than four liver metastases without demonstrable extrahepatic disease, where a tumour-free margin of at least 1 cm can be achieved. It is clear from published data that there is no place for incomplete resection of hepatic metastases as there is no survival benefit compared to patients who have not had resection (Scheele *et al.* 1995). The key role of imaging in patients considered for partial hepatectomy is to avoid an unnecessary laparotomy. Identification of a left lobe lesion in a patient planned for right hepatectomy means that the operation will not be curative. In this case surgery may be abandoned or the operation modified to local wedge resection of two or three lesions. It is here that the detection of subcentimetre lesions becomes of great importance. Intra-operative ultrasound with higher resolution than transabdominal scanning has a high sensitivity and has been shown to identify lesions missed with all other modalities pre-operatively (Soyer *et al.* 1993; Rafaelsen *et al.* 1996). It is best used in conjunction with systematic inspection and palpation of the liver, as small capsular and subcapsular lesions may be missed (Leen 1996). Laparoscopy has been shown to have an advantage for the detection of some sub-centimetre lesions, particularly, peripheral lesions and peritoneal seeding on the liver capsule (Rahusen *et al.* 1999). Currently, CTAP remains the most sensitive generally available imaging technique and, when combined with lesion targeted, high-resolution ultrasound, provides an acceptable accuracy for pre-operative assessment of resectability (Seltzer & Holman 1989; Karl *et al.* 1993).

However, if we are to increase the percentage of long-term survivors or true curative resection, the value of pre-operative imaging must be assessed on more than comparative sensitivity. Most comparative studies are flawed as they are cross-sectional, looking only at detected metastases rather than outcome or follow-up to identify those patients who later develop metastases. Leen *et al.* (1996) showed that IOUS failed to detect occult disease in 22 out of 27 patients with apparently curative resection of the primary tumour, who subsequently developed hepatic involvement (75 per cent of these within the first post-operative year).

Surgical planning requires evaluation of disease location with respect to segmental anatomy (Figure 10.4). MRI may have a more definite role here, both for improving the detection of small lesions and for defining anatomical relationships by multiplanar imaging in an easily recognisable format for the surgeon. An extended right hepatectomy will leave only segments 1, 2 and 3, and the volume of remaining liver should be at least 30 per cent of expected liver volume (Sugarbaker 1990). Since the presence of

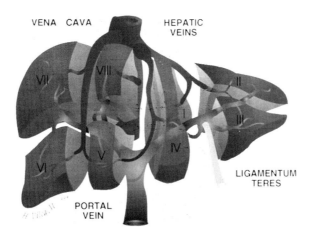

Figure 10.4 Segmental anatomy of the liver. Left lobe I –IV, right lobe V–VIII
Source: Reproduced with the kind permission of Dr Hector Vilca-Melendez.

underlying liver disease is a relative contraindication to surgery, radiological evidence of portal hypertension or cirrhosis may be an important additional finding on staging scans. Staging CT scans should be performed of the chest, abdomen and pelvis to exclude extrahepatic disease (Balthazar 1988; Zerhouni *et al.* 1996). Nodal involvement is the commonest site of extrahepatic disease – periportal, coeliac and para-aortic being the most frequent sites following resection of the primary tumour and regional nodes.

Where there is some question as to suitability for resection, a 'watch and wait' approach may be adopted. Given that disease progression must reflect the biology of the primary tumour, it is accepted that a patient who has developed no new lesions over a period of three months is unlikely to have occult lesions and may have a good chance of curative resection. If the patient is receiving adjuvant treatment in the hope of downstaging the disease, either with chemotherapy or local ablation therapy, a previously inoperable lesion may regress and re-evaluation may be indicated.

Post-operatively, a CT of the abdomen should be performed at one month as a new baseline. Disease recurrence may occur with the development of new lesions, presumably previously occult disease, or at the site of resection where the tumour-free margin may have been inadequate (Figure 10.5). Surveillance scanning should continue in these patients, initially at six-month intervals, as further resection or alternative therapies such as local ablation could be considered for isolated metastases with favourable tumour biology.

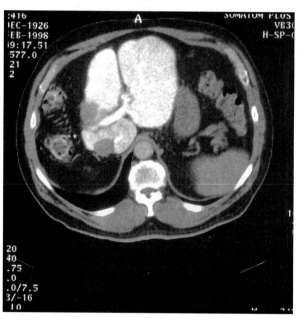

Figure 10. 5 Portal venous phase CT scan showing recurrence at the resection margin following right hepatectomy

Role of biopsy

Any lesion can be biopsied. Technical difficulty is seldom an issue. However, the aim of imaging should be to avoid the need for liver biopsy, which is associated with a considerable risk of haemorrhage and has an accepted mortality of one in 1,000. In addition to the risk of haemorrhage and more pertinent to this discussion, is the risk of tumour seeding along the needle track and to the peritoneum. When the diagnosis is in question, the true aim is to identify a metastatic deposit amenable to resection in a setting where there is a chance of prolonging survival and the potential to effect a cure. Any potential survival benefit would be jeopardised by the very high risk of tumour seeding (John & Garden 1993; Jourdan & Stubbs 1996).

Metastatic deposits represent the commonest cause of hepatic malignancy and are a common finding in general radiologic practice. The diagnosis is rarely difficult to make, especially if there is more than one lesion. Although the differential for a single lesion is wide, all other focal hepatic lesions have characteristic features such that with a lesion-targeted imaging approach, an accurate diagnosis is almost always possible. In the rare circumstance where the diagnosis remains in question, a 'watch and wait' approach should be adopted. The evolution and growth of a deposit will be evident, while any occult disease which would influence outcome following local resection will reveal itself, saving the patient an unnecessary laparotomy and allowing a more appropriate management decision to be made.

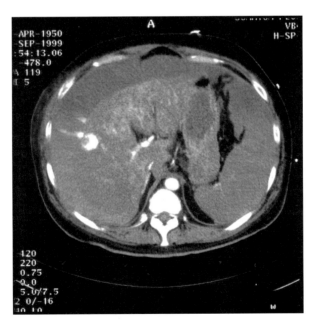

Figure 10.6 Complications of liver biopsy: CT scan following intravenous contrast shows profuse haemorrhage at the site of biopsy with a large haemoperitoneum

Recommendations

Staging of new primaries

- CXR
- Liver ultrasound
- Contrast-enhanced CT of the abdomen and pelvis

Surveillance post resection of primary

- Regular six-monthly liver ultrasound to 36 months
- Contrast-enhanced CT of the abdomen and pelvis at 12 months

Hepatic resection

- Helical CT, CTAP or MRI according to local facilities
- Laparoscopy with laparoscopic ultrasound may be advantageous prior to formal laparotomy
- Thoracic CT

Surveillance post-hepatic resection

- New 'baseline' scan at one month
- Six-monthly surveillance as for curative primary resection

Response to treatment (chemotherapy, tumour ablation)

- Three-monthly review with CT and/or ultrasound, aiming to keep radiation dose to a minimum

Biopsy

- A multimodality approach to characterising a solitary liver lesion should include ultrasound, dual-phase CT, tissue-specific contrast-enhanced MRI and angiography
- Biopsy should be avoided owing to the high risk of tumour seeding in a patient with the potential for curative partial hepatectomy

References

Adson MA (1983). Hepatic metastases in perspective. *American Journal of Roentgenology* **140**, 695–700.

Balfe DM (1992). Hepatic metastases from colorectal cancer: radiologic strategies for improved selection [editorial; comment]. *Radiology* **185**, 18–19

Bartolozzi C, Lencioni R, Ricci P, Paolicchi A, Rossi P & Passariello R (1998). Hepatocellular carcinoma treatment with percutaneous ethanol injection: evaluation with contrast-enhanced color Doppler US. *Radiology* **209**, 387–393

Bellin MF, Zaim S, Auberton E, Sarfati G, Duron JJ, Khayat D & Grellet J (1994). Liver metastases: safety and efficacy of detection with superparamagnetic iron oxide in MR imaging [see comments]. *Radiology* **193**, 657–63

Blomley MJ, Albrecht T, Cosgrove DO, Patel N, Jayaram V, Butler-Barnes J, Eckersley RJ, Bauer A & Schlief R (1999). Improved imaging of liver metastases with stimulated acoustic emission in the late phase of enhancement with the US contrast agent SH U 508A: early experience. *Radiology* **210**, 409–16

Carter R, Hemingway D, Cooke TG, Pickard R, Poon FW, McKillop JA & McArdle CS (1996). A prospective study of six methods for detection of hepatic colorectal metastases. *Annals of The Royal College of Surgeons of England* **78**, 27–30

Ch'en IY, Katz DS, Jeffrey RB Jr, Daniel BL, Li KC, Beaulieu CF, Mindelzun RE, Yao D & Olcott EW (1997). Do arterial phase helical CT images improve detection or characterization of colorectal liver metastases? *Journal of Computer Assisted Tomography* **21**, 391–7

Delbeke D (1999). Oncological applications of FDG PET imaging. *Journal of Nuclear Medicine* **40**, 1706–15.

Divgi CR, McDermott K, Griffin TW, Johnson DK, Schnobrich KE, Fallone PS, Scott AM, Hilton S, Cohen AM & Larson SM (1993). Lesion-by-lesion comparison of computerized tomography and indium-111-labeled monoclonal antibody C110 radioimmunoscintigraphy in colorectal carcinoma: a multicenter trial. *Journal of Nuclear Medicine* **34**, 1656–61

Fong Y, Saldinger PF, Akhurst T *et al.* (1999). Utility of 1BF-FDG positron emission tomography scanning on selection of patients for resection of hepatic colorectal metastases. *American Journal of Surgery* **178**, 282–87.

Fowler RC, Harris KM, Swift SE, Ward M & Greenwood DC (1998). Hepatic Doppler perfusion index: measurement in nine healthy volunteers. *Radiology* **209**, 867–71

Hagspiel KD, Neidl KF, Eichenberger AC, Weder W & Marincek B (1995). Detection of liver metastases: comparison of superparamagnetic iron oxide-enhanced and unenhanced MR imaging at 1.5 T with dynamic CT, intraoperative US, and percutaneous US. *Radiology* **196**, 471–8

Hemingway DM, Cooke TG, McCurrach G, Bessent RG, Carter R, McKillop JH & McArdle CS (1992). Clinical correlation of high activity dynamic hepatic scintigraphy in patients with colorectal cancer. *British Journal of Cancer* **65**, 781–2

Hollett MD, Jeffrey RB, Jr., Nino-Murcia M, Jorgensen MJ & Harris DP (1995). Dual-phase helical CT of the liver: value of arterial phase scans in the detection of small (≤1.5 cm) malignant hepatic neoplasms. *AJR American Journal of Roentgenology* **164**, 879–84

John TG & Garden OJ (1993). Needle track seeding of primary and secondary liver carcinoma after percutaneous liver biopsy. *HPB Surgery* **6**, 199–203; discussion 203–4. Review.

Jourdan JL & Stubbs RS (1996). Percutaneous biopsy of operable liver lesions: is it necessary or advisable? *New Zealand Medical Journal* **109**, 469–70

Kan Z, Ivancev K, Lunderquist A, McCuskey PA, Wright KC, Wallace S & McCuskey RS (1993). In vivo microscopy of hepatic tumors in animal models: a dynamic investigation of blood supply to hepatic metastases. *Radiology* **187**, 621–6

Kane PA, Ayton V, Walters HL, Benjamin I, Heaton ND, Williams R & Karani JB (1997). MnDPDP-enhanced MR imaging of the liver. Correlation with surgical findings [see comments]. *Acta Radiologica* **38**, 650–4

Karl RC, Morse SS, Halpert RD & Clark RA (1993). Preoperative evaluation of patients for liver resection. Appropriate CT imaging [see comments]. *Annals of Surgery* **217**, 226–32

Knol JA, Marn CS, Francis IR, Rubin JM, Bromberg J, Chang AE, Scheele J, Stang R, Altendorf-Hofmann A & Paul M (1993). Comparisons of dynamic infusion and delayed computed tomography, intraoperative ultrasound, and palpation in the diagnosis of liver metastases. Resection of colorectal liver metastases. *American Journal of Surgery* **165**, 81–7

Kuszyk BS, Bluemke DA, Urban BA, Choti MA, Hruban RH, Sitzmann JV & Fishman EK (1996). Portal-phase contrast-enhanced helical CT for the detection of malignant hepatic tumors: sensitivity based on comparison with intraoperative and pathologic findings. *AJR American Journal of Roentgenology* **166**, 91–5

Leen E, Angerson WJ, Wotherspoon H, Moule B, Cook TG & McArdle CS (1995). Detection of colorectal liver metastases: comparison of laparotomy, CT, US, and Doppler perfusion index and evaluation of postoperative follow-up results [see comments]. *Radiology* **195**, 113–16

Leen E, Angerson WJ, O'Gorman P, Cooke TG & McArdle CS (1996). Intraoperative ultrasound in colorectal cancer patients undergoing apparently curative surgery: correlation with two year follow-up. *Clinical Radiology* **51**, 157–9

Leveson SH, Wiggins PA, Giles GR, Parkin A & Robinson PJ (1985). Deranged liver blood flow patterns in the detection of liver metastases. *British Journal of Surgery* **72**, 128–30

Nelson RC, Thompson GH, Chezmar JL, Harned RK 2nd & Fernandez MP (1992). CT during arterial portography: diagnostic pitfalls. *Radiographics* **12**, 705–18; discussion 719–20.

Oppo K, Leen E, Angerson WJ, Cooke TG & McArdle CS (1998). Doppler perfusion index: an interobserver and intraobserver reproducibility study. *Radiology* **208**, 453–7

Paul MA, Blomjous JG, Cuesta MA & Meijer S (1996). Prognostic value of negative intraoperative ultrasonography in primary colorectal cancer. *British Journal of Surgery* **83**, 1741–3

Platt JF, Francis IR, Ellis JH & Reige KA (1997). Liver metastases: early detection based on abnormal contrast material enhancement at dual-phase helical CT [see comments]. *Radiology* **205**, 49–53

Rafaelsen SR, Kronborg O, Fenger C & Drue H (1996). Comparison of two techniques of transrectal ultrasonography for the assessment of local extent of polypoid tumours of the rectum. *International Journal of Colorectal Diseases* **11**, 183–6

Rahusen FD, Cuesta MA, Borgstein PJ, Bleichrodt RP, Barkhof F, Doesburg T & Meijer S (1999). Selection of patients for resection of colorectal metastases to the liver using diagnostic laparoscopy and laparoscopic ultrasonography. *Annals of Surgery* **230**, 31–7.

Scheele J, Stangl R & Altendorf-Hofmann A (1990). Hepatic metastases from colorectal carcinoma: impact of surgical resection on the natural history. *British Journal of Surgery* **77**, 1241–6

Seltzer SE & Holman BL (1989). Imaging hepatic metastases from colorectal carcinoma: identification of candidates for partial hepatectomy. *AJR American Journal of Roentgenology* **152**, 917–23

Semelka RC, Worawattanakul S, Kelekis NL, John G, Woosley JT, Graham M & Cance WG (1997). Liver lesion detection, characterization, and effect on patient management: comparison of single-phase spiral CT and current MR techniques. *Journal of Magnetic Resonance Imaging* **7**, 1040–7

Semelka RC, Cance WG, Marcos HB & Mauro MA (1999). Liver metastases: comparison of current MR techniques and spiral CT during arterial portography for detection in 20 surgically staged cases *Radiology* **213**, 86–91

Seneterre E, Taourel P, Bouvier Y, Pradel J, Van Beers B, Daures JP, Pringot J, Mathieu D & Bruel JM. (1996). Detection of hepatic metastases: ferumoxides-enhanced MR imaging versus unenhanced MR imaging and CT during arterial portography. *Radiology* **200**, 785–92.

Soyer P, Levesque M, Elias D, Zeitoun G & Roche A (1992). Preoperative assessment of resectability of hepatic metastases from colonic carcinoma: CT portography vs sonography and dynamic CT. *AJR American Journal of Roentgenology* **159**, 741–4

Soyer P, Elias D, Zeitoun G, Roche A & Levesque M (1993). Surgical treatment of hepatic metastases: impact of intraoperative sonography. *AJR American Journal of Roentgenology* **160**, 511–14

Sugarbaker PH (1990). Surgical decision making for large bowel cancer metastatic to the liver. *Radiology* **174**, 621–6

Sugarbaker PH (1999). Repeat hepatectomy for colorectal metastases. *Journal of Hepatobiliary Pancreatic Surgery* **6**, 30–8

Tsao JI, Loftus JP, Nagorney DM, Adson MA & Ilstrup DM (1994). Trends in morbidity and mortality of hepatic resection for malignancy. A matched comparative analysis. *Annals of Surgery* **220**, 199–205.

Valls C, Lopez E, Guma A, Gil M, Sanchez A, Andia E, Serra J, Moreno V & Figueras J (1998). Helical CT versus CT arterial portography in the detection of hepatic metastasis of colorectal carcinoma. *AJR American Journal of Roentgenology* **170**, 1341–7

Ward J, Naik KS, Guthrie JA, Wilson D & Robinson PJ (1999). Hepatic lesion detection: comparison of MR imaging after the administration of superparamagnetic iron oxide with dual-phase CT by using alternative-free response receiver operating characteristic analysis. *Radiology* **210**, 459–66

Weg N, Scheer MR & Gabor MP (1998). Liver lesions: improved detection with dual-detector-array CT and routine 2.5-mm thin collimation [see comments]. *Radiology* **209**, 417–26

Wernecke K, Rummeney E, Bongartz G, Vasallo P, Kivelitz D, Wiesmann W, Peters P, Reers B, Reiser M & Pircher W. Detection of hepatic masses in patients with carcinoma: comparative sensitivities of sonography, CT and MR imaging. *American Journal of Roentgenology* **157**, 731–9.

Zerhouni EA, Rutter C, Hamilton SR, Balfe DM, Megibow AJ, Francis IR, Moss AA, Heiken JP, Tempany CM, Aisen AM, Weinreb JC, Gatsonis C & McNeil BJ (1996). CT and MR imaging in the staging of colorectal carcinoma: report of the Radiology Diagnostic Oncology Group II. *Radiology* **200**, 443–51

Chapter 11

Image-guided percutaneous ablation of colorectal liver metastases

William R Lees and Alison R Gillams

Non-surgical ablation of liver metastases

Of the 28,000 new cases of colorectal cancer presenting each year in the UK, over half will develop liver metastases. The majority of these will be of limited number with systemic metastases being a secondary phenomenon. This is the rationale behind surgical resection, which, although never proven in a randomised controlled trial, yields five year survival of 20–45 per cent in carefully selected patients (Scheele *et al.* 1996; Scheele & Altendorf-Hofman 1998). Few patients with colon cancer are screened for liver metastases with other than an annual ultrasound scan and hence relatively few patients in the UK are diagnosed early enough to benefit from hepatic resection. With the recent focus on poor survival figures in the UK compared with the rest of Europe, this is now changing and most colorectal tumour boards are proposing screening with six monthly spiral CT for all patients for up to two years. It is very unusual for a metastasis to appear after this time if the screening scans are of good quality.

Despite the presence of metastases in other parts of the body liver metastases are the cause of death in many patients with colon cancer. The tumour volume doubling time is typically 100 days in our practice but a very wide range of behaviour is observed, with volume doubling times as short as two weeks. If detected sufficiently early and treated effectively a large proportion of patients are curable.

Surgical resection has until recently been the only therapy to realise this potential but few patients will be suitable for resection. Reasons for rejection include extrahepatic disease, site or number of metastases within the liver, unfitness for major surgery, age or unwillingness to accept the associated morbidity.

Because of these factors there has been strong interest in developing methods of local tumour ablation that can be applied either intra-operatively or percutaneously using image guidance (Solbiati 1998; Cuschieri 1999; de-Jode 1999).

Methods of ablation

The last ten years has seen the development of many ways of destroying tissue in situ. There are essentially three techniques: thermal ablation, direct injection chemotherapy and irradiation.

Thermal methods of tumour ablation

- High powered focused ultrasound
- Microwaves
- Interstitial laser photocoagulation
- Radiofrequency ablation
- Cryotherapy

Direct injection treatments

- Ethanol
- Taxol
- Cisplatin and other standard chemotherapeutic agents
- Gene therapy

Other methods

- Laser based photodynamic therapy
- Radioactive seed implants
- Interstitial radiotherapy

Properties of colorectal liver metastases affecting choice of therapy

In order to grow within the liver, a metastasis must parasitise its blood supply from the surrounding normal vascular bed. The new vascular circulation that develops within the metastasis is chaotic and disordered compared with the surrounding normal liver vessels. It shows arteriovenous connections, numerous blind-ending vessels and lacks vasomotor tonal regulation. The tumour environment is generally hypoxic and the abnormal vascular endothelium coupled with an absence of lymphatics leads to a high transport of water from the vascular bed into the surrounding extra-cellular fluid compartment raising the pressure within the tumour compared to that of the surrounding normal liver. Water flows from the tumour to the periphery producing peri-tumoural oedema up to the region where the excess water is carried away by the lymphatics of the normal liver tissue (Feldmann *et al.* 1997; Vaupel 1997).

The vast majority of metastases are hypovascular compared to the surrounding liver. Measurements in my laboratory using dynamic CT methods have shown that the typical colorectal carcinoma metastasis has a perfusion of approximately 0.2 mls/ml/minute which is comparable to the arterial component of perfusion in the normal liver. Metastases from other primaries such as breast show even less perfusion. It is only metastases from neuro-endocrine tumours that show significant hypervascularity.

The high water content of colorectal metastases increases the volume of the extra-cellular fluid compartment to in excess of 50 per cent of the tumour mass.

This leads to a low density appearance on unenhanced CT and the pure arterial supply means that the metastasis will be optimally identified during the portal venous phase of a multiphasic CT scan.

Colorectal metastases are rarely spherical. They are often partly necrotic and frequently grow by combination of radial expansion, venous invasion and budding. It has been known for many years from the surgical literature that there is almost always tumour in the surrounding normal liver which cannot be visualised by imaging techniques. Surgical teaching is that a centimetre margin of normal liver should be removed along with the tumour and that local recurrence rates are high if the margins are less than 5 mm (Taylor *et al.* 1997).

With all thermal ablation techniques, it is a common finding that the relatively low perfusion of the metastasis allows heat conduction to the margin of an even irregularly shaped tumour but that it is difficult to get adequate margins beyond this (Goldberg *et al.* 1998). Thirty to sixty per cent of colorectal metastases show a hypervascular rim. The nature of this perfusion abnormality has been debated for many years, but it has been consistently demonstrated with contrast enhanced ultrasound, dynamic CT, MRI with several contrast agents and by FDG PET. The PET data suggests that most of the active tumour metabolism takes place within this rim. The classical surgical teaching that a one centimetre margin is needed is supported by this known tumour biology (Smith *et al.* 1988; Wang 1992; Gerard *et al.* 1999; Miles *et al.*1999).

In addition to this tumour phenomenon, dynamic perfusion CT measurements at the time of treatment under CT guidance have shown that there is an immediate vaso-dilatory response of the normal hepatic arterial circuit in response to thermal injury. Arterial perfusion changes from 0.2–1.2 ml/ml/minute, actively cooling down the normal liver tissue. Large vessels in the vicinity of tumours also act as heat sinks and small amounts of tumour are often preserved in these regions. It is not surprising that even though a lesion can appear completely ablated on CT or MRI criteria, relapse rates around the margins are high. These lead to the principle of continued treatment over time, with a few of our patients having as many as ten therapy sessions over periods of up to six years (Antin *et al.* 1993; Roberts *et al.* 1994).

Spiral CT is capable of detecting all colorectal metastases greater than 1cm in diameter. Smaller lesions can be detected but are difficult to characterise. MRI is definitely a slightly more sensitive technique, but spiral CT is cheaper and allows more effective comparisons over time with standardised techniques. After several ablation procedures it can be difficult to distinguish a healing response from new tumour and meticulous scanning technique is vital.

Percutaneous ethanol injection (PEI) therapy

Extensive work in Japan and Italy has shown that this is an effective method for treatment of small hepatocellular carcinomas. These tumours are soft, highly vascular and are surrounded by a hard shell of cirrhotic liver. This ensures that the injectate will diffuse uniformly throughout the tumour. Complete tumour destruction at a single treatment is unlikely unless large volumes of pure ethanol are used, but delivered in small doses repeatedly over several weeks it can be effective in destroying lesions up to 4 cm in diameter (Livraghi *et al.* 1995a and b; 1999).

The therapy can then be given on an outpatient basis. The main limitation to this technique is diffusion of the injectate out of the tumour onto the liver capsule and peritoneal surfaces which can be extremely painful. Large volumes of ethanol can be injected at a single session into lesions larger than 4 cm but general anaesthesia is then required (Livraghi *et al.* 1995b).

The results of this treatment method are now well established for small lesions with the survival of individual patients more dependent on the severity of the underlying cirrhosis than the stage of the hepatocellular carcinoma. There is also evidence that the technique is more effective when combined with arterial chemoembolisation.

Several groups have attempted to extend this treatment to liver metastases with very little success. A typical metastasis is hypovascular, hard and is surrounded by soft normal liver. The injectate will therefore spread poorly throughout the tumour and leak into the surrounding tissues. Spillage of ethanol onto the peritoneal surfaces causes significant pain and limits the total amount of ethanol that can be delivered into a colorectal metastasis at any single session (Amin *et al.* 1993; Becker *et al.* 1999).

Other direct injection therapies

Many other substances have been injected directly into tumours to produce local cell death. The most promising of these currently are chemotherapeutic agents such as cisplatin and anti-angiogenesis agents such as taxol. Thus far these therapies have been confined to early clinical trials and have yet to show significant local control rates.

Thermal ablation methods

Lasers, microwaves and radiofrequency electrodes are all capable of discharging thermal energy into tissues through percutaneous delivery systems. All produce the same bio-effect, namely coagulative necrosis.

The advantages of thermal ablation over direct injection methods are:

- Uniform necrosis within the heated area
- A low risk of bleeding complications in the coagulated region
- The protection of the vessels against damage as a result of blood flow in large vessels
- Self-sterilization. A temperature of 90° around the treatment device will kill most bacteria.
- The track can also be coagulated to prevent seeding metastases and capsular bleeding.

The disadvantages are:

- The size and shape of the coagulum is limited by blood flow in the tissues around the tumour and by the hyperaemic response of normal liver to thermal injury. Thus viable tumour can be preserved in the heat sink of a large vessel.
- Thermal damage to richly innervated structures (diaphragm, chest wall etc) induces pain lasting for up to 10 days after treatment.

All these devices rely on gentle 'cooking' to produce coagulative necrosis. Heat too quickly and the tissue will char leading to insulation of the delivery device and loss of the mechanical strength of the tissue. The heat flux therefore needs to be limited and to deposit useful amounts of energy it needs to be deposited over as large a volume as possible. This can be done in two ways: increasing the surface area of the probe by using multiple laser fibres or electrodes arrays; or by actively cooling the probe to reduce the heat flux locally at the surface of the electrode (Figure 11.1).

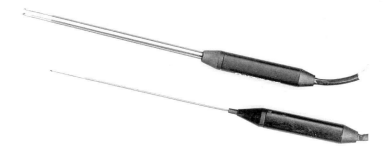

Figure 11.1 Single and triple cooled tip RF electrodes

A single application from any one of these devices can produce an area of necrosis up to 45 mm in diameter. With multiple applications, areas up to 7 or 8 cm can be achieved. The radiofrequency method using cooled tip cluster electrodes delivers the most power, allowing more rapid treatments or production of greater volumes of necrosis.

For colorectal cancer metastases the aim is to completely ablate the tumour and to produce a 1 cm margin of ablated normal liver (Figure 11.2) (Amin *et al.* 1993a, b and c; Solbiati *et al.* 1997; Goldberg *et al.* 1998; Vogl *et al.* 1998; Jiao *et al.* 1999; Torzilli *et al.* 1999; Dodd *et al.* 2000).

Because the major limiting factor in producing good marginal destruction of normal liver is the convection effect of blood flow there have been attempts recently to reduce hepatic arterial and portal venous blood flow. This has been achieved in three ways: balloon occlusion of the hepatic artery or portal vein (the radiological equivalent of the Pringle maneouvre; balloon occlusion of the draining lobar hepatic

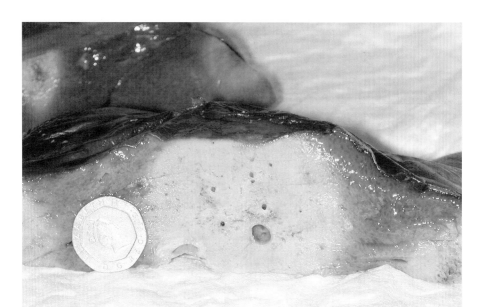

Figure 11.2 In vitro ablation. A 20 pence piece is 2 cm

vein; pharmacological manipulation and hypotensive anaesthesia. We use the latter method. All our patients undergo general anaesthesia and control of blood pressure is safe and easy to achieve. Known physiology indicates that a reduction in blood pressure of more than 30 per cent will reduce splanchnic blood flow by 50 per cent. The other methods also work but add risk or complexity to the procedure (Figure 11.3) (Goldberg *et al.* 1998).

Photo-dynamic therapy (PDT)

PDT uses light sensitive drugs (mainly porphyrin based) which are taken up by cells and when irradiated at specific wavelengths destroy the target tissue by free radical production. For some tumours there is a degree of selective concentration for many of the agents used. Tissue destruction is achieved at very low powers (fractions of a Watt) so that no thermal damage is produced. There is no destruction of collagen within the treated tissue hence in theory its mechanical strength is not lost.

The major disadvantage is that for the more effective agents currently available clearance from the body is very slow and the patients must avoid daylight for up to ten days.

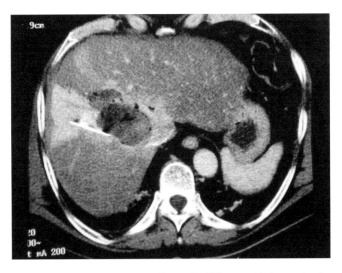

Figure 11.3 Immediate post-treatment dynamic CT scan. Note marked perfusion changes in associated normal liver

With the very low powers used there are no immediately visible effects on US, CT or MRI. The full evolution of tissue damage takes several days so that the results of treatment can only be assessed by delayed scanning.

PDT has proven very successful for treating tumours of the skin, oro-pharynx and head and neck by surface illumination. We are now extending this technique to solid organs using multiple interstitial fibres running from solid state lasers operating at a wavlength specific to the PDT agent used, usually in the red part of the spectrum. At these wavelengths penetrance of the light is less than 1 cm and even using multiple fibres it is difficult to produce volumes of necrosis larger than 25 ml. This limits the applicability of this method in the liver where much larger volumes of necrosis are needed. We presently have experimental programs running for lung, pancreatic and prostate cancers.

Cryotherapy

Cryotherapy has been used for intra-operative ablation for nearly 20 years. Although of proven effectiveness the biggest series still contain relatively small numbers of patients. Volume of necrosis produced depends heavily on the size of the applicator and although percutaneous devices have been developed these produce only small volumes of necrosis in relatively long treatment times.

Imaging requirements for percutaneous treatment

Much is required of imaging in delivering percutaneous therapy. We must:

- Detect the metastases within the liver
- Map the distribution of the tumour in three dimensions
- Develop a treatment plan which will minimise collateral damage
- Determine a safe route to the target
- Guide the treatment device to the target point
- Observe the treatment effect
- Relate observed treatment effect to the ultimate bio-effect
- Determine completeness of treatment and modify delivery accordingly
- Follow the healing process
- Detect recurrence

Guidance and delivery systems

Ultrasound is not particularly effective at detecting colorectal metastases. They are often isoechoic and are freqently situated in areas difficult to visualise such as high beneath the dome of the diaphragm or in a lateral subcapsular position. This will change with development of new contrast agents for ultrasound but no systematic data is yet available.

Helical CT used with iodinated contrast is capable of detecting all colorectal metastases greater than 1 cm in diameter and is currently our recommended technique for detection. Most lesions will only be seen during the portal venous phase of contrast opacification which is of no use for guidance. In the equilibrium phase when iodinated contrast has passed from the blood pool to the extracellular fluid compartment lesion conspicuity is poor.

MRI has the advantage of excellent detection capabilities and with the use of long acting liver specific contrast agents can also be used for guidance. The major disadvantage is cost and limited availability (Vogl *et al.* 1998; de Jode *et al.* 1999).

Using ultrasound or CT guidance it is possible to direct a needle into any target that can be clearly visualized. Ultrasound guidance has the advantage of speed and the ability to track moving structures. CT has the advantage of greater geometric precision. We now use a combination of the two methods for most of our solid organ treatments. Dynamic contrast enhanced CT is also the method of choice for evaluating the effect of treatment. Successful tissue necrosis will produce complete tissue devascularization which is seen at CT as non-enhancement after injection of IV contrast. The effects visualized by ultrasound are too subtle to accurately assess necrosis, although contrast enhanced Doppler methods show promise. We have shown by animal experiments that the area of devascularisation seen at CT corresponds to the ultimate necrosis to within 1–2 mm.

MRI is the only imaging method that has the theoretical capability to provide all the information described above.

Interventional MR systems are now available at 0.2–0.5 Tesla which, although highly effective, deliver poor quality images at rapid scan times (1–5 seconds) compared to the high field strength systems used for diagnosis.

MRI can also be combined with 3-dimensional optical tracking devices to deliver true frameless stereotaxis. It is possible to drive the scanner to produce freehand images in near real time just like an ultrasound machine.

MR techniques are developing rapidly. High field strength interventional systems capable of 'fluoroscopic' MR imaging are being constructed and will be available within two years.

Results of ablation therapies in colorectal metastases

Outcome of therapy can be measured by technical success, tumour free interval and by survival. The concept of technical success can be assessed for individual metastases but requires follow up of at least six months to be sure that a metastasis has been completely ablated. Incomplete ablation does not necessarily mean failure, although it does indicate the need for further treatment. In our own database, of tumours that were thought to be completely ablated at the 18 hour CT scan 36 per cent had recurred locally by a mean of 8.5 months (Figures 11.4 and 11.5).

Tumour free interval is an imprecise measure and depends heavily on screening interval and the quality of the imaging studies used. Our data does show that prognosis is better if a patient is rendered apparently tumour free than if there is any residual tumour.

Survival time is the definitive end point. It is only in the past year that the pioneering groups working in tumour ablation have been producing reliable survival data extending to four and five years. Even there, the early results are not as good as

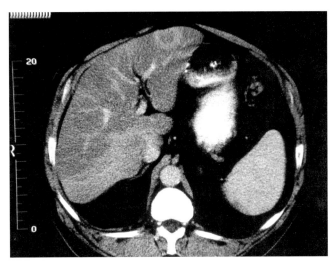

Figure 11.4 Two colorectal metastases pre-ablation

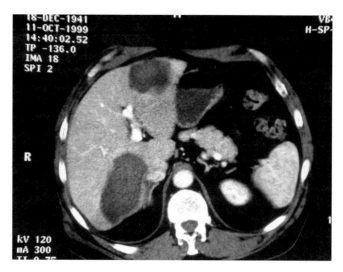

Figure 11.5 Eighteen hour post-ablation CT. Complete ablation plus margins

more recent ones because of continuous technical improvement, a better understanding of the tumour biology and a more aggressive approach to therapy.

Using a cooled tip laser under MRI guidance, Vogl has reported a median survival for over 200 patients with colorectal metastases of 39.3 months with local complete ablation rates of 68 per cent. Solbiati has produced similar figures for radiofrequency ablation but with a shorter follow up.

We performed multifibre laser ablation until 1998. Since then we have used single and triple cluster cooled tip radiofrequency devices with a 200W generator. These are capable of producing large volumes of necrosis in relatively short treatment times, typically 30–45 minutes. It is now entirely feasible to produce a confluent volume of necrosis of up to 300 ml (9 cm diameter) in treatment times of less than one hour.

Our most recent figures (combined laser and RF data) for survival of 109 patients with colorectal metastases show a median survival of 49 months for those who fit our strict selection criteria of fewer than five metastases with a maximum lesion size of 6 cm. Those patients who fall outside these criteria have a median survival of 24 months.

These figures compare very favourably with the surgical data which reports five year survival of 20-50 per cent.

Most of the difference between the ablation series can be ascribed to selection bias (Figure 11.6).

There is an obvious need for a randomised controlled trial of ablation, first compared with surgery using surgical acceptance criteria but allowing early crossover with surgical resection of incompletely treated lesions at RF and RF of surgical recurrence. Modelling using data from our surgical and our RF database suggests that an optimal strategy combines both approaches.

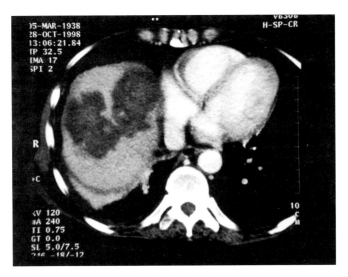

Figure 11.6 Two areas of ablation after treatment scanned at one month with dynamic CT. No enhancement is seen in the ablated area

The issues which tax us at the present time are: how to produce the largest possible volume of necrosis; how to minimise collateral damage and hence complications and how vigorously to continue to treat patients with limited disease that we fail to eradicate completely at our initial treatment sessions.

Quality of life issues dominate discussion about these therapies. We presently perform all our RF ablations of liver tumours under general anaesthesia. We use hypotensive anaesthesia to reduce both portal venous and hepatic arteial blood flow to minimise local convection. Post-procedural pain is well controlled by steroids or NSAIDs.

The more aggressive we have become with treatment, the more complications we have seen. Since January 1995, we have treated 797 liver metastases in 141 patients, with a mean age of 62 years (range 33-87). Cooled tip RF resulted in 501 mets in 64 patients during 127 treatment sessions; interstitial laser resulted in 296 mets in 77 patients during 340 treatment sessions.

These figures reflect the improvement in treatment efficiency. More metastases were treated in more patients at fewer treatment sessions. The technique continues to improve leading to a change in acceptance criteria.

From diagnosis of liver metastases our median survival in the optimal group (strict accordance with acceptance criteria) is a median of 49 months. For those outside these ctriteria the median survival is 24 months.

Optimal group;

1 year	98%
2 year	89%
3 year	70%
4 year	51%

From time of first ablation therapy, which typically would be after failure of first line chemotherapy, the medial survival in the optimal group is 32 months.

We have experienced one fatality in this time due to sepsis secondary to malignant biliary obstruction. We have had five cases of segmental liver infarction none of which have been clinically significant. There have been five abscesses. Three of these have been secondary infection of liver necrosis after systemic sepsis. One was an RF burn between liver and colon. All were successfully managed with systemic antibiotics and percutaneous drainage. All five took at least two months to heal.

Multiple liver punctures will lead to bleeding complications. Unsurprisingly we had five significant subcapsular haematomas. Only one required transfusion. Pleural effusions and right basal consolidation are common but are symptomatic only in patients with poor pulmonary reserve. Post-procedural pain is seen in 10–15 per cent of RF patients but is usually well controlled with oral analgesia and anti-inflammatory drugs. Ninety-eight per cent of our patients are discharged from the hospital within 24 hours of treatment.

Do we influence the survival of patients with colorectal liver metastases? This remains to be proven in a randomised controlled trial. A randomised controlled trial has never been performed for surgical resection of colorectal liver metastases. Our results in patients who are unsuitable for resection are comparable to those of many published surgical series. The advent of percutaneous image-guided ablative therapy will provoke a new look at treatment for colorectal liver metastases.

Possible randomised controlled trials include RF versus surgery in an operable group (allowing early crossover for relapse after either technique) and chemotherapy with and without RF.

References

Amin Z, Bown SG, Lees WR (1993a). Local treatment of colorectal liver metastases: A comparison of interstitial laser photocoagulation (ILP) and percutaneous alcohol injection (PAI). *Clinical Radiology* **48**, 166–71.

Amin Z, Bown SG, Lees WR (1993b). Liver tumour ablation by interstitial laser photocoagulation: Review of experimental and clinical studies. *Seminars in Interventional Radiology* **10**, 88–100.

Amin Z, Donald JJ, Masters A *et al.* (1993). Hepatic metastases: interstitial laser photocoagulation with real-time US monitoring and dynamic CT evaluation of treatment. *Radiology* **187**, 339–47.

Amin Z, Harris SA, Lees WR, Bown SG (1993). Interstitial tumour photocoagulation. *Endoscopic Surgery and Allied Technology* **1**, 224–9.

Antin Z, Thurrell W, Spencer GM *et al.* (1993). Computed tomography-pathologic assessment of laser-induced necrosis in rat liver. *Invest-Radiology* **28**, 1148–54.

Becker D, Hansler JM, Strobel D, Hahn EG (1999). Percutaneous ethanol injection and radio-frequency ablation for the treatment of nonresectable colorectal liver metastases – techniques and results. *Langenbecks Archives of Surgery* **384**, 339–43.

Cuschieri A, Bracken J, Boni-L (1999). Initial experience with laparoscopic ultrasound-guided radiofrequency thermal ablation of hepatic tumours. *Endoscopy* **31**, 318–21.

de-Jode MG, Lamb GM, Thomas HC, Taylor-Robinson SD, Gedroyc-WM (1999). MRI guidance of infra-red laser liver tumour ablations, utilising an open MRI configuration system: technique and early progress. *Journal of Hepatology* **31**, 347–53.

Dodd GD III, Soulen MC, Kane RA *et al.* (2000). Minimally invasive treatment of malignant hepatic tumors: at the threshold of a major breakthrough. *Radiographics* **20**, 9–27.

Feldmann HJ, Molls M, Vaupel P (1997). Blood flow and oxygenation status of human tumors. Clinical investigations. *Klin Padiatr* **209**, 243–9.

Gerard A, Pector JC, Bleiberg H (1999). Hepatic artery ligation or embolization and locoregional chemotherapy of liver metastases from colorectal cancer. *Strahlenther Onkol* **175**, 1–9.

Goldberg SN, Hahn PF, Halpern EF, Fogle RM, Gazelle GS (1998). Radio-frequency tissue ablation: effect of pharmacologic modulation of blood flow on coagulation diameter. *Radiology* **209**, 761–7.

Gillams AR & Lees WR (2000). Survival after image guided percutaneous ablation of colorectal liver metastases. *Dis Colon & Rectum* **43**(5), 656–62.

Goldberg SN, Hahn PF, Tanabe KK *et al.* (1998). Percutaneous radiofrequency tissue ablation: does perfusion-mediated tissue cooling limit coagulation necrosis? *Journal of Vascular Interventional Radiology* **9**, 101–11.

Goldberg SN, Solbiati L, Hahn PF *et al.* (1998). Large-volume tissue ablation with radio frequency by using a clustered, internally cooled electrode technique: laboratory and clinical experience in liver metastases. *Radiology* **209**, 371–9.

Jiao LR, Hansen PD, Havlik R, Mitry RR, Pignatelli M, Habib N (1999). Clinical short-term results of radiofrequency ablation in primary and secondary liver tumors. *American Journal of Surgery* **177**, 303–6.

Livraghi T, Bolondi L, Buscarini L *et al.* (1995). No treatment, resection and ethanol injection in hepatocellular carcinoma: a retrospective analysis of survival in 391 patients with cirrhosis. Italian Cooperative HCC Study Group. *Hepatology* **22**, 522–6.

Livraghi T, Giorgio A, Marin G *et al.* (1995). Hepatocellular carcinoma and cirrhosis in 746 patients: long-term results of percutaneous ethanol injection. *Radiology* **197**, 101–8.

Livraghi T, Goldberg SN, Lazzaroni S, Meloni F, Solbiati L, Gazelle GS (1999). Small hepatocellular carcinoma: treatment with radio-frequency ablation versus ethanol injection. *Radiology* **210**, 655–61.

Miles KA, Leggett DA, Kelley BB, Hayball MP, Sinnatamby R, Bunce I (1999). In vivo assessment of neovascularization of liver metastases using perfusion CT. *Langenbecks Arch Surg* **384**, 313–27.

Roberts HR, Paley M, Hall-Craggs MA *et al.* (1994). Dynamic magnetic resonance control of interstitial laser photocoagulation therapy of colorectal hepatic metastases (letter) *Lancet* **343**, 1221.

Scheele J & Altendorf-Hofmann A (1998). Resection of colorectal liver metastases. *Langenbecks Arch Surg* **384**(4), 313–27. **415**, 1–31.

Scheele J, Altendorf-Hofmann A, Stangl R, Schmidt K (1996). Surgical resection of colorectal liver metastases: Gold standard for solitary and radically resectable lesions. *Swiss-Surg* **4**, 4–17.

Smith FW, Heys SD, Evans NT *et al.* (1988). Pattern of 2-deoxy-2-[18F]-fluro-D-glucose accumulation in liver tumours:primary, metastatic and after chemotherapy. *Gan To Kagaku Ryoho* **15**, 2351–4.

Solbiati L (1998). New applications of ultrasonography: interventional ultrasound. *European Journal of Radiology* **27**, 200–6.

Solbiati L, Goldberg SN, Ierace T *et al.* (1997). Hepatic metastases: percutaneous radio-frequency ablation with cooled-tip electrodes. *Radiology* **205**, 367–73.

Taylor M, Forster J, Langer B, Taylor BR, Greig PD, Mahut C (1997). A study of prognostic factors for hepatic resection for colorectal metastases. *American Journal of Surgery* **173**, 467–71.

Torzilli G, Livraghi T, Olivari N (1999). Interstitial percutaneous therapies in primary and secondary liver tumors. *Ann Ital Chir* **70**, 185–94.

Vaupel PW (1999). The influence of tumor blood flow and microenvironmental factors on the efficacy of radiation, drugs and localized hyperthermia. *Klin Padiatr* **209**(4), 243–9.

Vogl TJ, Mack MG, Muller PK, Straub R, Engelmann K, Eichler K (1999). Interventional MR: interstitial therapy. *European Radiology* **9**, 1479–87.

Vogl TJ, Mack MG, Roggan A *et al.* (1998). Internally cooled power laser for MR-guided interstitial laser-induced thermotherapy of liver lesions: initial clinical results. *Radiology* **209**, 381–5.

Wang C (1992) Mangafodipir trisodium (MnDPDP)-enhanced magnetic resonance imaging of the liver and pancreas. *Nucl Med Commun* **13**, 193–5.

Chapter 12

Unresectable hepatic metastases from colorectal cancer: longterm remission through chemotherapy combined with surgery

René Adam, Eli Avisar, Arie Ariche, Daniel Azoulay, Denis Castaing, Sylvie Giachetti, Francis Kunstlinger, Francis Levi and Henri Bismuth

Introduction

Colorectal cancer commonly spreads to the liver. It is estimated that approximately 50 per cent of patients with colorectal tumours will fail in the liver at some point in the course of the disease (Steele & Ravikumar 1989), while 15–20 per cent of the patients will also have liver disease at presentation (Fong *et al.* 1996). In almost one third of cases, the liver was shown at autopsy to be the only site of cancer spread (Weiss *et al.* 1986). This finding supports the concept of liver resection or other means of antineoplastic therapy to the liver as a potentially curative treatment. Hepatic resection for colorectal metastases results in 20–45 per cent five-year survival (Adson *et al.* 1984; Fortner *et al.* 1984; Hughes *et al.* 1988; Nordlinger *et al.* 1992; Scheele *et al.* 1995; Fong *et al.* 1997), however, only 10–20 per cent of patients presenting with liver metastases are amenable to curative resection (Adson 1987; Doci *et al.* 1991; Bismuth *et al.* 1996). Palliative and symptomatic treatment is commonly offered to the rest of the patients and median survival does not exceed 15 months. Over the past eight years, our unit has managed these patients in a protocol of neoadjuvant chemotherapy. Using a multidisciplinary approach, liver resection has been routinely reconsidered in all the cases of objective response to the treatment. This chapter reviews our results with this approach.

Patients and methods

All the patients with colorectal liver metastases who presented to Paul Brousse Hospital from February 1988 to September 1996 were entered into a prospective non-randomised study. Upon initial evaluation the patients were divided in two groups according to resectability of the liver disease. Patients with resectable disease were scheduled for surgery. The non-resectable group was treated with a neoadjuvant chemotherapy protocol, with resectability of the lesions periodically reconsidered according to tumour response. As previously reported (Bismuth *et al.* 1996), we classified the non-resectable lesions into four categories: large size, ill location, multinodularity and extrahepatic disease.

Patients were mainly treated with intravenous chronomodulated chemotherapy combining 5-fluorouracil (5-FU) (700–1,200 mg/m²/day), folinic acid (300 mg/m²/day) and oxaliplatin (25 mg/m²/day). Previously, the patients could have received, elsewhere, as many as seven different chemotherapy regimens with no response sufficient to reconsider surgery. Every course lasted four to five days, with intervals of two to three weeks in between courses. The treatment was administered in an ambulatory setting via a time/dose multi-channel pump. The rationale for this technique, which has been described by Levi *et al.* (1992), is to optimise dose intensities and drug tolerance by means of a treatment which is modulated in a sinusoidal fashion along a 24-hour period with peak flow rates at 04.00 hours for 5-FU and folinic acid, and at 16.00 hours for oxaliplatin. Evaluation by ultrasound for objective response was performed every three treatments by the same radiologists. Biochemical criteria of response included decreased carcino-embryonic antigen (CEA) and CA 19-9 levels. Reconsideration for resection followed each evaluation. The criteria for surgery consisted in the feasibility of a curative resection, be it in one or two stages, coupled with a plateau in the response to chemotherapy. Different surgical techniques were used to enable the resection, including portal vein embolisation to hypertrophy the remaining liver, as described by Azoulay *et al.* (1995), two-stage resections when all the lesions could not be resected by a single procedure, and cryotherapy or radiofrequency, usually combined with surgery, to allow a complete treatment of tumours, in patients otherwise unresectable. All the surgically treated patients after neoadjuvant chemotherapy received additional chemotherapy according to the same protocol for six months after the resection. The treatment was then discontinued in patients with no evidence of disease and normal tumour markers. Follow-up was performed every three months with physical examination, ultrasound, CEA and CA19-9. In addition, a CT scan of the chest and abdomen was performed every six months. Recurrent disease was treated according to the same protocol again, with re-operation when feasible, or chemotherapy. All the demographic, clinical, surgical, radiological and biochemical patient's information was entered in a database which served to assess the results of our treatment. Survival curves were calculated according to Kaplan Meier actuarial survival technique.

Results

Eight hundred and seventy-two patients were entered in this study: 171 (19.6 per cent) had a curative resection, and the remaining 701 were considered non-resectable and treated with our protocol of neoadjuvant chemotherapy. Ninety-five of these 701 patients achieved a measurable response to the neoadjuvant treatment and subsequently underwent a potentially curative resection (13.5 per cent) (Figure 12.1). These patients received 3 to 29 courses of chemotherapy (mean=10), during 3–29 months (mean=10.6). An objective reduction in tumour size following chemotherapy was observed in all patients subsequently submitted to liver resection. A significant

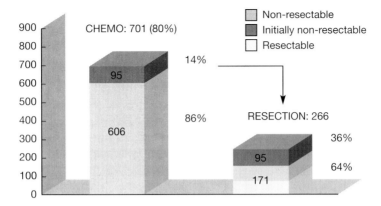

Figure 12.1 Colorectal liver metastases: 827 patients (Paul Brousse Hospital, 1988–1996)

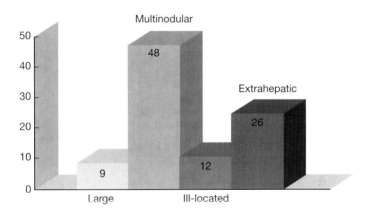

Figure 12.2 Cause of initial non-resectability – 95 patients resected after chemotherapy

reduction of tumour markers was also demonstrated (mean CEA levels from 190 (1–4,225) to 47 ng/ml (1–1,243) and CA 19-9 levels from 4,477 (22–228,000) to 219 IU/ml (2–5,900). The initial cause of unresectability was either large size (n=9), or bad location (n=12), or multinodularity (n=48) or presence of extrahepatic disease (n=26) (Figure 12.2). More than one hepatectomy was required in 28 patients, and portal vein embolisation or ligation was performed in five patients. All visible extrahepatic disease was resected at the same time or during a second operation. These associated procedures included pulmonary resections (20), splenectomy (1), nephrectomy (1), oophorectomy (3), adrenalectomy (1), lymphadenectomy (3), resection of colonic recurrence (2) and partial resection of the diaphragm (2). There was no peri-operative mortality during the first 60 days after surgery. Twenty-two (23 per cent) complications were recorded, two post-operative hemorrhages requiring a laparotomy, four infected and eight sterile fluid collections treated non-operatively, four transient biliary fistulas and four systemic complications.

After a mean follow-up of 4.2 years (range 1.3–9.9), 39/95 patients are alive (41 per cent). Twenty-five of these patients have no evidence of disease (26 per cent) (Figure 12.3). The overall five-year survival for the post-neoadjuvant resection group is 34 per cent (Figure 12.4).

When divided by the different non-resectability categories five-year survival is 60 per cent for large lesions, 49 per cent for ill-located tumours, 37 per cent for multinodular disease and 18 per cent for extrahepatic disease (Figure 12.5).

Discussion

Surgical resection is the only effective treatment for hepatic metastases of colorectal cancer. However, this option is available only to a minority of patients. For the majority, where surgery is not a curative option, palliative therapy only is available resulting in no long-term survivors (Hughes *et al.* 1988). The reasons for unresectability can be divided into two categories: diffuse extrahepatic disease, which would not be controlled by treatment of the liver disease, and intrahepatic disease, which would endanger the patient's life if resected. No available form of systemic therapy can effectively eradicate diffuse metastatic disease but a partial response to chemotherapy could be used to downstage the liver disease, which would then be amenable to surgical resection. In a selected number of cases the same logic can be applied to a limited amount of extrahepatic disease, which could then be resected also. The combination of 5-FU folinic acid and oxaliplatin has recently been

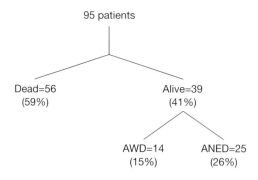

Figure 12.3 Current patients' status (95 patients). (AWD = alive with disease; ANED = alive with no evidence of disease)

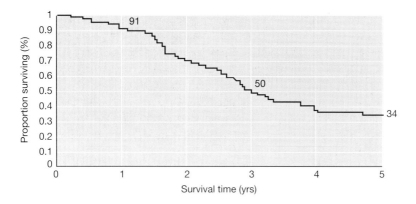

Figure 12.4 Five-year survival of liver resection after systemic chronotherapy (95 patients)

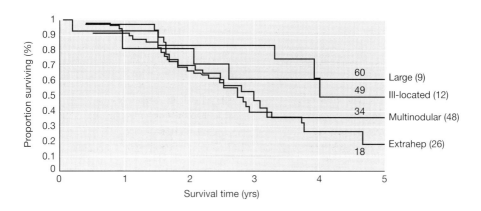

Figure 12.5 Five-year survival of liver resection after systemic chronotherapy for the different categories of non-resectability

shown to have a response rate of 59 per cent. Oxaliplatin is a recently developed platinum compound with no nephrotoxicity and a good activity against colorectal tumours (Becouarn *et al.* 1997). Chronomodulation of the therapy enables the delivery of higher concentrations of these agents with a higher tolerance rate and fewer complications than flat therapy (Levi *et al.* 1995; Bertheault-Cvitkovic *et al.* 1996; Levi *et al.* 1999). The most significant decrease in complications is with the occurrence of severe stomatitis, which was shown in a randomised trial to drop from 89 to 18 per cent (Levi *et al.* 1994). In another multicentre trial, chronotherapy reduced fivefold the rate of severe mucosal toxicity, halved the incidence of functional impairment from peripheral sensory neuropathy and increased the response rate from 29 per cent to 51 per cent (Levi *et al.* 1997).

Our results with neoadjuvant chemotherapy for colorectal liver metastases were previously published for a smaller number of patients and a shorter follow-up (Bismuth *et al.* 1996). In this series there was a 13.5 per cent rate of conversion from unresectability to resectability with a curative potential. This number would have been higher if we had excluded patients treated with second- or third-line chemotherapy for whom the chance of subsequent surgery is more remote than with first-line treatment. If calculated for the whole group of 872 patients, neoadjuvant chemotherapy was able to increase the initial tumour resectability rate from 19.6 per cent to 30.5 per cent. This increased number of curative resections was accompanied by a 'reasonable' complication rate and a five-year survival rate similar to that for initially resectable lesions. In addition, these figures concern an overall population of patients with hepatic metastases, irrespective of the presence of extrahepatic tumour and of the type of neoadjuvant chemotherapy. Five-year survival was close to 50 per cent in the patients whose metastatic disease was confined to the liver and who received chronomodulated 5-FU, folinic acid and oxaliplatin (Giachetti *et al.* 1999).

As expected, because of the nature of the disease, patients with multinodular lesions had a worse prognosis than those with large or ill-located tumours. In addition, they were more likely to require more than one operation and additional procedures, such as portal vein embolisation or cryotherapy. Patients with extrahepatic disease had a five-year survival of 18 per cent only and merely 2/26 patients remained disease-free. These results would support a greater selectivity in aggressively resecting patients with extrahepatic disease.

In conclusion, major hepatic resections after tumour response to chemotherapy can provide a source of hope for long-term survival. Further analysis is required to define the subset of unresectable patients which is most likely to benefit from resection in the long term.

References

Adson MA, Van Heerden JA, Adson MH *et al.* (1984). Resection of hepatic metastases from colorectal cancer. *Archives of Surgery* **119**, 647–51.

Adson MA (1987). Resection of liver metastases. When is it worthwhile? *World Journal of Surgery* **11**, 511–20.

Azoulay D, Raccuia JS, Castaing D *et al.* (1995). Right portal vein embolization in preparation for major hepatic resection. *Journal of The American College of Surgeons* **181**, 267–9.

Becouarn Y, Ychou M, Ducreux M *et al.* (1997). Oxalatplatin (L-OHP) as first line chemotherapy in metastatic colorectal cancer (MRC) patients: preliminary activity/toxicity report. *Proceedings of the American Society of Clinical Oncology* **16**, (abstr. 804).

Bertheault-Cvitkovic F, Jami A *et al.* (1996). Bi-weekly itensified ambulatory chronomodulated chemotherapy with oxaloplatin, 5-fluorouracil and folinic acid in patients with metastatic colorectal cancer. *Journal of Clinical Oncology* **14**, 2950–8.

Bismuth H, Adam R, Levi F *et al.* (1996). Resection of nonresectable liver metastases from colorectal cancer after neoadjuvant chemotherapy. *Annals of Surgery* **224**, 509–22.

Doci R, Gennari L, Bignami P *et al.* (1991). One hundred patients with hepatic metastases from colorectal cancer treated by resection: Analysis of prognostic determinants. *British Journal of Surgery* **78**, 797–801.

Fong Y, Kemeny N, Paty P *et al.* (1996). Treatment of colorectal cancer hepatic metastasis. *Seminars in Surgical Oncology* **12**, 219–52.

Fong Y, Cohen A, Fortner JG *et al.* (1997). Liver resection for colorectal metastases. *Journal of Clinical Oncology* **15**, 938–46.

Fortner JG, Silva JS, Golbey RB *et al.* (1984). Multi-variate analysis of a personal series of 247 consecutive patients with liver metastases from colorectal cancer. *Annals of Surgery* **199**, 306–16.

Giachetti S, Itzhaki M, Gruia G *et al.* (1999). Long term survival of patients with unresectable colorectal cancer liver metastases following infusional chemotherapy with 5-fluorouracil, leucovorin, oxaliplatin and surgery. *Annals of Oncology* **10**, 663–9.

Hughes KS, Simon R, Songhorabodi S *et al.* (1988). Resection of the liver for colorectal carcinoma metastases: a multi-institutional study of indications for resection. *Surgery* **103**, 278–88.

Levi F, Misset JL, Brienza S *et al.* (1992). A chronopharmacologic phase II clinical trial with 5-fluorouracil, folinic acid and oxaliplatin using an ambulatory multichannel programmable pump. *Cancer* **69**, 893–900.

Levi F, Giacchetti S, Adam R *et al.* (1995). Chronomodulation of chemotherapy against metastatic colorectal cancer. *European Journal of Cancer* **31**A, 1264–70.

Levi F, Zidani R, Brienza S *et al.* (1999). A multicenter evaluation of intensified ambulatory chronomodulated chemotherapy with oxaliplatin, 5-fluorouracil and leucovorin as initial treatment of patients with metastatic colorectal carcinoma. *Cancer* **85**, 2532–40.

Levi F, Zidani R, Vannetzel JM *et al.* (1994). Chronomodulated versus fixed-infusion-rate delivery of ambulatory chemotherapy with oxaliplatin, fluorouracil and folinic acid (leucovorin) in patients with colorectal cancer metastases: a randomized multi-institutional trial. *Journal of the National Institute of Cancer* **86**, 1808–17.

Levi F, Zidani R, Misset JL *et al.* (1997). Randomised multicentre trial of chronotherapy with oxaliplatin, fluorouracil, and folinic acid in metastatic colorectal cancer. *Lancet* **350**, 681–8.

Nordlinger B, Jaeck D, Guiguet M *et al.* (1992). *Traitement des metastases hepatiques des cancers colorectaux. Monographies de l'Association Francaise de Chirurgie (AFC).* Paris (France), Springer Verlag (pp.129–46).

Scheele J, Stang R, Altendorf-Hofmann A *et al.* (1995). Resection of colorectal liver metastases. *World Journal of Surgery* **19**, 59–71.

Steele G Jr & Ravikumar TS (1989). Resection of hepatic metastases from colorectal cancer: biologic perspectives. *Annals of Surgery* **210**, 127–38.

Weiss L, Grundmann E, Torhorst J *et al.* (1986). Hematogenous metastatic patterns in colonic carcinoma: an analysis of 1541 necropsies. *Journal of Pathology* **150**, 195–203.

Index